The
Impatient Woman's Guide
to Getting Pregnant

The
Impatient Woman's Guide
to Getting Pregnant

Jean M. Twenge, Ph.D.

ATRIA PAPERBACK

New York   London   Toronto   Sydney   New Delhi

ATRIA PAPERBACK
A Division of Simon & Schuster, Inc.
1230 Avenue of the Americas
New York, NY 10020

This Atria Paperback edition February 2013

ATRIA PAPERBACK and colophon are trademarks of
Simon & Schuster, Inc.

For information about special discounts for bulk purchases,
please contact Simon & Schuster Special Sales at 1-866-506-1949
or business@simonandschuster.com.

The Simon & Schuster Speakers Bureau can bring authors to your live event.
For more information or to book an event, contact the Simon & Schuster
Speakers Bureau at 1-866-248-3049 or visit our website
at www.simonspeakers.com.

DESIGNED BY ERICH HOBBING

Manufactured in the United States of America

10 9 8 7 6 5

The Library of Congress has cataloged the Free Press edition as follows:
    Twenge, Jean M.
    The impatient woman's guide to getting pregnant/Jean M. Twenge.
        p. cm.
    Includes index.
    1. Conception—Popular works. 2. Pregnancy—Popular works. I. Title.
    RG133.T84 2012
    618.2—dc23
    2011031050

ISBN 978-1-4516-2070-2
ISBN 978-1-4516-2071-9 (ebook)

To my children

Contents

Foreword   ix

Introduction   xiii

1: What to Do Before You Start Trying   1

2: Supplements, Exercise, and the SOS Diet   33

3: Not the Kind of Egg That Comes in a Carton:
How to Figure Out When You Are Ovulating   52

4: Horizontal Mambo: The Best Time to Dance
the Baby Dance   75

5: Choosing the Sex of Your Baby   85

6: Not as Scary as You've Heard: The Real Stats on
Age and Fertility   102

7: "If One More Person Tells Me to 'Just Relax' . . .":
The Psychological Side of Getting Pregnant   116

8: Peeing on More Sticks: The Two-Week Wait and
When to Test for Pregnancy   140

9: Sad Endings: Miscarriage   153

10: When to See Your Doctor and What to Expect
When You Do   165

11: Congratulations, and Get Ready to Go to Bed at
8pm: After You're Pregnant   177

Contents

Appendix A: The Really Impatient Woman's
Guide to Getting Pregnant: Most of the Advice,
All of the Truth, with a Few of the Jokes   183

Appendix B: Abbreviations Decoded: How to
Acronym with the Rest of the Crowd   185

Appendix C: Countdown to Trying   187

Appendix D: The Impatient Woman's Shopping
List   190

Appendix E: Food Ideas   192

Appendix F: Troubleshooting   195

Appendix G: More Details on Having a Girl or
a Boy: How Shettles Got It Wrong   198

Appendix H: Further Reading   203

References   205

Acknowledgments   217

Index   221

Foreword

By Sarah M. Appleton, M.D.
Department of Obstetrics and Gynecology,
University of Colorado Hospital

When I tell people I am an obstetrician and gynecologist,
I am often met with a series of responses, one of which is
usually "You must love working in such a *happy* field." True.
There is nothing more amazing than helping to welcome a
family's new addition into the world. However, most people do not recognize the anxiety that many of my patients
face even before conception.

Deciding to start a family can be overwhelming. Further, it is an intimate subject, and often women would
rather discuss their concerns with their close girlfriends or
sisters. Alas, their best buddies may not have all the facts
or know how to interpret the confusing data and statistics
repeated throughout the media. This is where *The Impatient
Woman's Guide to Getting Pregnant* comes in. Dr. Twenge
reviews the important details about preparing and trying to
conceive with a thorough review of the literature, a healthy
dose of humor, and the familiarity of a friend.

You may have already read that you need to start taking

prenatal vitamins even before trying to conceive, but you have probably also read confusing or contradictory information on other vitamins and supplements, diet, exercise, timing of conception, home monitoring kits, and more. There are few resources available to patients that review the medical evidence reliably. With her expertise in research, Dr. Twenge interprets the data regarding natural conception for her readers while presenting the information in a way that is easy to understand.

As a provider who also sees patients dealing with depression and anxiety during and after pregnancy, I have seen the effects trying to conceive can have on mental health. Stress and anxiety commonly affect patients and their partners. Without an effective plan to manage these feelings, couples can feel isolated from loved ones and frustrated with the process. Certainly, the frequent colloquial advice of "just relax" is ineffective and infuriating to those wanting to get pregnant. In *The Impatient Woman's Guide to Getting Pregnant*, a variety of stress-reduction techniques and healthy coping mechanisms are reviewed, many of which I encourage my patients to use.

On a busy day in my clinic, I met Diana*, a new patient scheduled for a "PCC" visit—Preconception Counseling. Like many of my patients, Diana was a planner. As an adolescent, she selected her university early. From college, she went straight to law school, applied to the "right" internships at the best law firms and worked hard—all the way to a partnership in the firm. Along the way, she met her

* A pseudonym

husband; as expected, he is also a planner. After establishing much of their lives, they were now ready to start their family. They sat before me with questions I had heard frequently in the office:

Can I get pregnant?

What do I need to do before we start trying?

Am I healthy enough for pregnancy?

Is our life too stressful for pregnancy?

What can we do to improve our chances of conceiving?

Can we control anything about the process?

What if we don't get pregnant in three months? Six months? One year?

Did we wait too long?

Ultimately, Diana, her husband, and I had a long discussion to answer their questions and set up a plan of action. I am hopeful they left my office with their apprehensions reduced and with a positive outlook about taking the next steps in expanding their family. Similarly, *The Impatient Woman's Guide to Getting Pregnant* is a resource that successfully provides answers to questions, eases concerns, and offers hope to its readers.

So, if you are a woman who has planned the various elements in her life, and now you would like some guidance on how to improve your likelihood of getting pregnant, this book is for you. Maybe you aren't a planner, but you want to play an active role in your fertility, then this book is for you. Or perhaps you just have questions about trying to conceive, and you want to get helpful information with a dose of humor and realism, then read on!

Introduction

Okay, you admit it: You're an Impatient Woman. Maybe you've planned your career and are now ready to start a family with the same organized, well-informed approach. Or maybe you've been trying to get pregnant for a few months, which is enough to make any woman Impatient. Perhaps you're a little older and don't have time to be casual about your fertility. Maybe you want to have a baby at a certain time of year due to career commitments, travel plans, or spacing your children apart. Or you don't want getting pregnant to take so long that you start to worry about your fertility. You might want to get pregnant quickly just so you can stop driving your husband nuts. (Or your boyfriend or partner. For brevity, I'll use husband most of the time.)

When I was trying to conceive, I never found a book about getting pregnant that was fun to read, like talking to a girlfriend who knows a lot but also laughs a lot. Trying to get pregnant is not just medical—it's psychological, social, and sexual. It also involves an enormous amount of emotion, from anxiety and despair to hope and joy. Trying to conceive is alternately tragic and hilarious. Instead of cuddling after sex, you put pillows under your butt and sit with your legs in the air like an upturned insect. Two weeks later, you're squinting furiously at something you just peed on, praying for a second line to appear and feeling despondent when it doesn't. These experiences aren't just intercourse and urination; like many of the best events in life, they're comical and emotionally meaningful at the same time.

Books and websites by (usually male) fertility doctors can tell you about the latest tests, but there's a lot missing. How many of these doctors have woken their husbands for morning sex because they thought they were ovulating? How many have nervously peed on a stick at 5am because they couldn't wait any longer or cried uncontrollably when their period came?

As for your husband—well, most guys are just not as impatient as we are, content to float along in their video-game and sports world, oblivious to the supreme importance of cervical mucus and stick-peeing. If men could get pregnant, there would probably be a lot more episodes of the show *I Didn't Know I Was Pregnant.* (Yes, this is a real TV show, complete with reenactments that usually culminate in a surprised woman giving birth on a toilet. A comedy program promptly relabeled the show *I Didn't Know I Had to Take a Dump.*)

You also deserve the most accurate information possible. When I was first trying to conceive, I read everything I could in books and online. I analyze data and write journal articles in my day job as a researcher, so I turned next to research studies published in medical journals. Over and over, I discovered that what I had found online, in books, and even on the instruction sheets for ovulation predictor kits was wrong, half wrong, or from a questionable source. My favorite example: The commonly mentioned statistic that a woman over 35 has only a 66 percent chance of getting pregnant within a year comes from a study of birth records from 17th-century France! Studies using more recent samples find much higher fertility for older women. Finding the real information based on actual studies helped me get pregnant fairly quickly despite being over 35 and having some fertility issues. Yet much of this scientifically rigorous and very helpful research isn't available where most women can find it. In these pages, I will share this exciting information with you.

I also noticed that most fertility books covered only part of the story. They'd discuss the physical aspects of getting pregnant without mentioning the emotional ones. They'd detail one method of ovulation prediction but leave out other methods. Or they'd go into exhausting detail about what to eat before trying to get pregnant but not cover much else. Perhaps because I'm an Impatient Woman, I wanted one book with all of this stuff instead of having to read 10 or 15. *The Impatient Woman's Guide to Getting Pregnant* is that book.

Some people, often middle-aged men, find the idea of a book about getting pregnant inherently funny: "I bet that's a short book—it just says, 'Have sex!' on every page." But of course it's more complicated than that. There are very good reasons to prepare for pregnancy and to learn as much as possible before you start trying. Women often want to get pregnant quickly, so it pays to know how to predict ovulation and the best time to have sex. You might even be able to tip the scales toward having a boy or a girl (though not in the way you may have heard; see Chapter 5). Some amazing research shows that what you consume before your baby is born—from food to vitamins to alcohol—influences your child's health and intelligence. The brain and nervous system start developing incredibly early, around two weeks after conception. When you've prepared to get pregnant, you're more likely to give your baby the best start in life.

Trying to get pregnant is very emotional and stressful because ultimately it's out of our control. In an age of reliable birth control, we can now consciously decide to try to get pregnant. This gives us the illusion that getting pregnant is controllable. There are plenty of things you can do to increase your odds—and I will tell you about as many of those as possible—but getting pregnant is partly based on luck, internal body mechanisms, and other uncontrollable factors. It also involves an infuriating amount of waiting. If you're an Impatient Woman, this is extremely difficult, even if you've only been trying for a few months. As a psychologist, I can share coping strategies based on the latest research. As a woman who has gone through the stress of trying to get pregnant three times (four if you count my early miscarriage), I've also experienced the strong emotions that no amount of training can prepare you for.

Anxiety about fertility can begin even before you start trying to get pregnant. Courtney*, for example, is only 20,

---

*A pseudonym, as are the names of all the women whose stories are included in the book. In addition, in some instances identifying details have been changed.

but says, "I've always dreamed of having kids and fear that something will keep me from having my own biological children. I really don't want to have kids for about another five years. Still, my fertility is something I worry about." Then ramp up that anxiety when you're actually trying, and when you've been trying for three months, and then six months, and it's easy to understand why trying to get pregnant can really freak you out. The key is to strike a balance between learning a lot and becoming completely obsessed. I'll tell you how to distract yourself so that you're not thinking about fertility every second, and I'll share some techniques for combating anxiety and depression naturally. Here are two you can start right now: Take a supplement of 1,000 milligrams of fish oil a day and learn the relaxation technique of deep breathing. When you're not stressed, practice closing your eyes and breathing deeply. If you then do this when you're stressed, your body will get the message to calm down and you will start to feel better.

Because this book is *not* called *The Patient Woman's Guide . . .* , it is fairly short. If you're a Really Impatient Woman, check out Appendix A for the very quick summary of advice. (I'm still working on the version for Really, Really Impatient Women, which will fit on a Post-it note.) I list the research studies in the References section at the end of the book, so you can read the original research if you're as crazy as I am. Did I say crazy? I meant curious.

This book is primarily about natural conception—what you can do in your own bedroom (or kitchen or favorite hotel room) to get pregnant quickly and maybe even influence the sex of your child. I'll cover the difficult decision of deciding when to see a fertility specialist and what you can expect from your initial visit, but not the more involved fertility treatments such as in vitro fertilization (IVF). However, I will mention many research studies done on women undergoing IVF—mostly because they're the population most often studied by fertility researchers.

Enjoy the months when you're trying to get pregnant. That advice is much easier to give than it is to take. We are so used to being able to control everything and obtaining instant results. Getting pregnant defies those expectations. Even if you get pregnant the first month, you still have to wait two weeks to ovulate and almost two weeks to find out. Read this book, talk to your friends, and do what you can, but realize there's fun in it, too. You're about to start your trying to conceive (TTC) journey. Enjoy the ride.

CHAPTER 1

What to Do Before
You Start Trying

Not long ago, women who wanted to get pregnant simply threw away their birth control and went about their
lives. Few knew anything about when they ovulated or gave
much thought to how their diet might affect their fertility.
The idea of preparing to get pregnant would have seemed
strange.

Not anymore. These days, more and more women take
a proactive approach. We're Impatient Women (IWs for
short, because we're very busy) who don't want to sit around
and wait. We're organized and achievement driven—that's
how we got into college or got a good job or planned our
wedding—so we take that same goal-oriented approach to
building a family. We're also anxious about infertility. We've
heard about couples who struggled for years to get pregnant and we're afraid that will be us. Some of us are in our
thirties or forties and don't have any time to waste.

There are many benefits to planning and preparing for
your pregnancy. One study found that most women feel
no symptoms of pregnancy until 20 days after ovulation—
at least a week after pregnancy tests become reliable. The

embryo's heart and nervous system are already developing then and are most vulnerable to the effects of alcohol, tobacco, prescription drugs, and other things that could cause birth defects. Folate, the B vitamin that drastically reduces the risk of neural tube birth defects, is most effective if it's taken *before* conception. So by planning ahead and testing for pregnancy early (though not too early! See Chapter 8), you're not tempting fate or thinking too much—you're just practicing being a mother, protecting your children before they're even conceived.

But be prepared to hear that you should "just relax," the two words guaranteed to make an IW roll her eyes. When I asked Allison, 38, if her mother had a different perspective on trying to conceive, she said, "Oh, yeah. How annoying is that? My girlfriends and I always talk about how our mothers say, 'We never even knew about tracking ovulation or any of that. You just need to relax. Stop worrying about it so much.'" Although it's true that worrying all the time is no way to live (more on that later), taking prenatal vitamins and planning to get pregnant isn't worrying too much. It's just plain smart.

Vice Taxes

If politicians start talking about taxing it when there's a budget crisis, you shouldn't be doing it when you're trying to get pregnant. That means cigarettes, drugs, alcohol, and even caffeine. All are linked to fertility problems, miscarriage, or birth defects, especially at higher levels of consumption. It's fine to drink a little (a glass or two of wine with dinner on the weekends) before you ovulate and up to six days afterward (the earliest an embryo can implant). After that, you should lock up the fun juice for a week or so. Then you will either get a negative pregnancy test, which is an excellent excuse to raid the booze cabinet (though not too much), or you will get a positive pregnancy test, which means your Two-Buck-Chuck is going to take a nine-month-long vacation. Most studies suggest that light to moderate drinking (less than two drinks per day) doesn't harm fertility, but more than three drinks per day ups the risk of infertility to 60 percent. Interestingly, men's heavy drinking negatively affects fertility even more than women's heavy drinking.

Smoking and drugs should be eliminated at least three months before trying so that your body can rid itself of the toxins. Smoking sharply increases the risk of infertility and even causes women to go into menopause earlier. But the effects of smoking dissipate fairly rapidly after quitting. Other drugs such as marijuana take longer to leave the body, primarily because THC, the active chemical in pot, gets stored in fat cells. If you or your partner are having trouble quitting smoking or drugs or cutting down on drinking, ask your primary care doctor for advice. There are lots of options for treatment.

I've saved the dearest for last: caffeine. Your Grande Skim Latte Extra Foam—or more precisely, the caffeine in it—is a drug. Yes, I know: That's why it's so awesome. Unfortunately, studies show a link between excess caffeine (two or more cups of coffee a day) and taking longer to get pregnant. Moderate to high caffeine intake is also related to miscarriage. Nonsmoking women who consumed between 300 and 699 milligrams of caffeine a day (about two to five cups of coffee) cut their fertility by 12 percent, and those who consumed more than 700 milligrams cut it by more than a third. The effect on men's fertility was even more severe, with those drinking five or more cups of coffee a day cutting their fertility in half. So you and your guy can keep going to Starbucks, but only once a day. If you need more caffeine, consider getting it from tea (especially green tea, which has other health benefits), as some studies have found that tea can help fertility.

Or consider doing something radical like getting enough sleep so that you don't need so much caffeine. Sleep deprivation buzzkills everything from mood to the immune system. Most adults need at least seven hours, and eight is better. Sleeping this much is *not* a waste of time; it's a biological imperative for good health. Also, get some sun exposure without sunscreen for 15 to 30 minutes (depending on the season) a few times a week in the middle of the day (between 10am and 2pm), especially in the spring, summer, and fall. Sunlight on your skin generates vitamin D, which has been linked to better fertility and lots of other health benefits. The book *The Vitamin D Solution* has much more on this; vitamin D from sunlight stays in your body longer than supplements, and you can't overdose on it. Sunlight also helps you sleep better. (The book also explains that it's fine to get a little sun exposure without sunscreen.)

Lifestyle factors have a big effect on fertility. One study found that couples with four or more bad habits (such as smoking, heavy caffeine intake, and heavy drinking) took an amazing *seven times* longer to get pregnant. This is actually good news: It means you can significantly boost your fertility by factors you can control. As one friend put it, "When you're trying to get pregnant, confine your bad habits to messiness, pornography, and shoplifting." Because men have to change their habits too, you might have some convincing to do. Promising more sex in place of less beer might work. And then, just when you've gotten him to heave the Heineken, you have an even bigger job: Convincing him to have his ejaculate analyzed. This one might take all of your wifely powers.

A Semen Analysis for Your Partner

Up to half of fertility problems are caused by sperm issues (the technical term is *male factor*, which sounds like a really bad men's cologne). Because men always have it easier, tests for sperm issues are quick and inexpensive—between $50 and $100 at a doctor's office. (There are home kits, too, but they are less accurate and more expensive. Most test sperm count but not motility or form, which are just as important.) Insurance usually doesn't pay for a semen analysis, but it's a fairly small amount of money for some very helpful information. Try to talk your husband into having a semen analysis before you start trying to get pregnant. If the news is good, as it's likely to be, you will have eliminated the possibility of about 40 percent of fertility issues. If it's not good, he can see a fertility doctor or a urologist as soon as possible. Sperm issues can often be solved through common and relatively inexpensive techniques such as intrauterine insemination (IUI) or outpatient surgery for varicoceles (a problem with blood flow in the testicles). Other times, a short course of antibiotics can clear up sperm problems.

Kendall, who got pregnant with her first child fairly quickly, tried for a year to get pregnant again. She and her husband went through all of the expensive infertility tests, and she was distressed to learn she had low egg supply at age 37. But the tests yielded another surprise: signs of bacterial infection in her husband's semen sample (just a regular infection, not a sexually transmitted one). Kendall and her husband took a round of antibiotics, and a few months later Kendall was pregnant. Not all sperm issues will respond this quickly to treatment, of course, but Kendall's story illustrates the importance of getting a semen analysis as early as possible.

What if your husband doesn't like the idea of getting his sperm tested, especially if you haven't started trying to conceive yet? Remind him that spending 20 minutes buffing the banana with some soft porn is not so bad—after all, he voluntarily did this about three times a day when he was 14. Of course, it's not the self-pleasure that makes some men balk at the idea of a sperm analysis—it's performance anxiety. Men are often terrified that their sperm won't measure up and are thrilled when it does. My husband announced our first pregnancy to family members by saying, "My boys can swim," which just confused most of them. His brother liked to tell people he "slipped one past the goalie." My husband tried this one, too, until I reminded him that there was no goalie (more like somebody waving them in).

Try to take his perspective about the test. A sperm test is sexual, not just clinical like the fertility tests for women, and men's identities are very closely intertwined with their sexual prowess. Some men find it deeply embarrassing to hand over the cup at the doctor's office. The semen analysis issue can lead to some pretty serious fights—it's tough to be understanding when the test is so simple. One IW's husband said he found the test humiliating, which led to a huge fight in which she yelled, "Shut the f*** up and get your ass—actually, your penis—to the lab!"

If you admit to your partner that you're not just an Impatient Woman but also slightly nuts, it might help. If he's embarrassed to make the doctor's appointment, tell him that when he talks to the doctor he can always roll his eyes and say his wife is a little crazy. This is especially effective with a male doctor, who will probably laugh, say, "Yeah, mine, too," and hand over the lab slip.

Volunteer to go with him if it would make him more comfortable; ask the clinic just how much you're allowed to "help." Talk about what he'll do when he gets to the clinic: Is there anything in particular that he feels the most embarrassed or anxious about? And though you shouldn't poke fun at his feelings, you might have a good laugh coming up with fun porn titles he might watch (*Breast Side Story? Free My Willy? Ocean's Eleven Inches?*). You could tell him the nickname for the male sample room: the Spank Tank. Or you could tell hubby to imagine he's a donor at the Nobel Prize Sperm Bank—or, even better, its real name, the Repository for Germinal Choice.

IW Jenna employed a different strategy, shifting the

focus away from her husband by telling him to get the analysis done so that the doctor could move on to assessing *her* fertility. She also reminded him of all the other men they knew who'd done the test, making it seem more normal. In a particularly smart IW move, Jenna picked up the lab slip herself so that her husband wouldn't have to remember to schedule an appointment.

If you live close enough to a lab, your guy might be able to "provide" his sample in the comfort, privacy, and personal porn mag collection of his own home (or, if you can afford it, a hotel room close to the clinic). Semen samples have to get to the lab within 45 to 60 minutes of "collection" and must be kept warm during the journey. (Anyone want to put spooge down their shirt? In a plastic cup, fortunately.) If home is too far away, though, he'll have to do his snake charming at the lab, embarrassment included (though he can remind himself that the other guys are all there for the same thing).

If the sperm news isn't good, it can feel like a blow to your partner's masculinity. That's not surprising—many women feel just as deeply upset about their own fertility problems. It's like your body has betrayed you. But as Dr. Harry Fisch points out in his book *The Male Biological Clock*, "It's as ludicrous to blame oneself for a low sperm count or hormonal abnormality as it is to blame oneself for having impacted wisdom teeth or being color-blind." Remind your husband that this is just like a blood test or a urine test, and it's nothing to be embarrassed about. If a semen analysis produces an abnormal result, the test should be repeated a week or two later. Semen, like men, can have "bad" days—sperm counts can be low because of illness or for random reasons. So it's best to do the test twice—and if it's normal one of the two times, there's probably nothing to worry about.

Getting Your Guy Healthy . . . and Wearing the Right Underwear?

So what else can your guy do to speed things along? A lot of the same things that you're doing to get healthy—and preferably several months before you start trying, as men make sperm in 74-day cycles (that's about two and a half months). That means no smoking, no recreational drugs, and no heavy drinking or caffeine use. It's probably also a good idea for him to take a multivitamin. Make sure it includes vitamin E and zinc, both of which are important for sperm production.

Thankfully, briefs men don't have to become boxer men (or freeball men) when they're trying to become fathers—tighty whitey briefs don't adversely affect male fertility. Yes, there actually is a published study in the *Journal of Urology* titled "Are Boxer Shorts Really Better? A Critical Analysis of the Role of Underwear Type in Male Subfertility." The paper uses terms like *disordered testicular thermoregulation,* which has just the right connotation for the male anatomy being a finely tuned rocket. Despite the funny terms and topic, this was a well-designed experiment that looked at scrotal temperatures, sperm count, and lots of other variables, and showed that sperm count wasn't affected by underwear type. The study authors provide an interesting theory on why underwear type doesn't matter: "The supportive effect of brief type underwear of pulling the testes close to the body and lack of this effect with boxers is minimized by wearing pants. Therefore, unless one advocates wearing underwear alone or the abandonment of clothing altogether, advising infertility patients to wear a particular type of underwear appears to have little impact." In other words, the great equalizer in the underwear wars: the wonderful garment called pants. The coolest (pun intended) fact is that men would apparently achieve the best scrotal temperatures and thus maximum fertility by wearing skirts. Somehow I doubt that's going to happen.

Another study had 21 men wear polyester jockstraps, some with aluminum linings, for a year to see if it would affect sperm counts. It didn't, though how they got 21 guys to wear uncomfortable aluminum underwear for a year is beyond me. (And how did they make it through airport security? That would be an interesting pat-down from the TSA. "I swear, officer, I'm part of an experiment on metal underwear! Why don't you believe me?") Of course, a lot of women participate in uncomfortable underwear experiments every day. If you count underwire bras, we might even have the aluminum part covered.

Guys shouldn't spend too much time in hot tubs over 100°F, which can heat up the little guys too much and decrease sperm count, but not by a huge amount. Using a hot tub once a week or so is probably okay, but a conservative approach would be to avoid hot tubs for about three months before trying to conceive.

Seeing the Doctor Yourself

A lot of books recommend that you schedule a preconception visit with your doctor. I did, and when I told my doctor why I was there, she looked at me like I was crazy. It's just not the norm to see a doctor because you're merely *thinking* about getting pregnant. One approach is to frame the visit around what you need to get done—and there's a surprising number of things. For example, you'll want to get tested for infections, one of the most common causes of unexplained infertility.

It's also a good idea to get your immunizations updated. Childhood shots sometimes wear off, and diseases like rubella (sometimes called German measles) can cause birth defects if you have the bad luck to contract them when you're pregnant. It's not a good idea to get most immunizations when you're pregnant, so planning ahead is important. Ask your doctor if you can be tested for immunity to rubella. My immunity to rubella had worn off, so I got an MMR—measles, mumps, and rubella—shot before we started trying to get pregnant. Get a booster shot for DTaP (diphtheria, tetantus, and pertussis), and get vaccinated against chicken pox if you never had the shot or the disease. Having immunity to these diseases is important because many are becoming widespread again, probably due to decreased immunization rates. And get a flu shot every year (it's safe even if you are pregnant). Vaccinations are especially important if you work in a petri dish like a hospital or a school (some preschool teachers joke that their students are "viruses on legs").

You might also want to get your thyroid hormone levels checked. Low thyroid levels are surprisingly common among women—about 10 percent of us have them, and many don't know it. They're often caused by an autoimmune disorder called Hashimoto's thyroiditis (which sounds like it should be on a sushi menu). Low thyroid levels can cause irregular cycles, fertility issues, and problems during pregnancy. If it turns out that you have low levels, this is very treatable with replacement thyroid hormone in a prescription pill (including when you're pregnant). If you get the test, be sure to ask exactly what your TSH number is. If it's 3, that's borderline, and you might want to read up on thyroid issues before you talk to your doctor (just to be confusing, *high* TSH numbers mean *low* levels of thyroid hormone). Most labs don't flag a TSH result as abnormal until it's over 5 or 6, but some people experience symptoms even with levels of 3 or 4. Ideally, your TSH should be between 0.5 and 1.5 when you're trying to get pregnant.

If you have any medical conditions or regularly take any medications, you'll definitely want to ask about how getting pregnant will affect those. Some medications shouldn't be taken when you're pregnant or even trying to get pregnant, so you might need to find alternatives. And definitely schedule a dentist appointment. Gum infections and other dental problems are a potential cause of premature labor (weird but true), so it's good to be up to date on your dental care.

If you have serious concerns about your cycles—say, you have very irregular periods—a gynecologist will usually try to figure out the cause. For some women, the culprit is polycystic ovarian syndrome (PCOS), a disorder that often (but not always) co-occurs with being overweight. There are many fertility treatments for PCOS, including diet modifications and drugs. If you have a chronic health condition like diabetes, discuss your baby plans with your doctor.

If you have less serious concerns about your menstrual cycle, you might not get the answers you're looking for. Before I got pregnant the first time, I spotted for days and sometimes even a week before I got my period, which is clearly not normal. The nurse I saw had no advice for me and said weird cycles aren't a problem unless you've been trying to get pregnant for more than six months. I didn't like her overly blasé attitude, but it's true that the only way to know if you have a fertility problem is to try to get pregnant and see what happens. Impatient Women want the answer to a question doctors can't always answer: "Am I fertile?" Doctors don't want to do a lot of tests on you when there's a good chance you won't have any trouble getting pregnant. Most insurance plans won't pay for anything related to infertility. It's a frustrating situation, but they do have a point: Most women will be able to conceive naturally within a few months, so it's best to try first and not cry over milk that has yet to be spilled.

The tough thing is to stay sane during this time. Even before you start trying to get pregnant, it's natural to worry that it won't happen for you. That energy has to go somewhere, and for some women it goes into obsessing over their cycles, endlessly researching things online, and thinking about fertility during any spare moment. Psychologists call this pattern ruminating, and you will be happier if you try to avoid it. See Chapter 7 for advice on what to do instead.

Going Off Birth Control

If you've been using condoms or charting for birth control, you can start trying to conceive instantly—have unprotected sex on a fertile day, and boom, you're trying. If you've been using hormonal birth control, though, you'll have to plan ahead. Most doctors suggest having at least one normal cycle after birth-control pills (or other hormonal methods like the ring or patch) before you try to conceive, to make sure you go back to ovulating and have some time for your uterine lining to build back up (hormonal birth control can thin it out). Especially if you've been on the pill for years, it can take several cycles for your full fertility to return, so it's probably better to stop taking the pill at least three months, and maybe six months, before you start trying. In the meantime, you'll want to use condoms or chart (see Chapter 3).

Birth-control shots such as Depo-Provera can take longer to leave the body—up to nine months, which might cause irregular cycles during that time. So it's best not to get a Depo-Provera shot if you're thinking of getting pregnant within the next year. If you have an intrauterine device (IUD), you should be able to conceive shortly after it's removed, though it's a good idea to have one full cycle first just to let your uterus return to normal.

Environmental Hazards

Many of us spend our days in front of a computer screen. Fortunately, computer monitors won't affect your fertility. You might, though, want to take a look in your kitchen cabinets. Plastic can leach into food and deliver an unwanted dose of chemicals, which might affect fertility. Much attention has been focused on bisphenol-A (BPA), a chemical found in some soft plastics that mimics the hormone estrogen. One study found that women who had more BPA in their systems produced more unusable eggs during in vitro fertilization (IVF). BPA has not been studied in natural conception, but it's scary enough that you might want to consider the plastic in your house and how you use it. The usual advice is to make sure that the label on the plastic product says "BPA-free," and if it's recyclable, has a 2, 4, or 5 inside the recycling symbol (the others—1, 3, 6, and 7— are more likely to have BPA or other harmful stuff). Fortunately, most microwave meal containers are one of these safer plastics.

Chemicals are more likely to leach out of heated plastic, so if you cook rice, soup, or leftovers in your microwave, use a glass or ceramic container. Buy a stainless steel water bottle and drink most beverages in a real glass (they taste better that way, anyway). Don't use plastic wrap in the microwave. I do most of these things now, though I have not been able to find a vegetable steamer that's not plastic. The bigger problem is kids' stuff is almost all plastic, with good reason—giving a toddler a real glass results in an ER visit in an average of thirteen seconds.

If you work with chemicals in a lab, medical office, or dental office, you should thoroughly investigate any potential hazards. For example, dental assistants are exposed to X-rays and mercury in fillings, so you might have to adjust your work when you're trying to get pregnant.

Acupuncture and Herbs

Alternative medicine like acupuncture and natural supplements like herbs are extremely popular these days, especially among women who want to get pregnant. Even though lots of books and websites recommend acupuncture and herbs for fertility, there is very little actual research on them, and some of the research suggests they don't work.

Acupuncture doesn't seem to improve women's fertility, at least in IVF cycles. Initially, a few small studies suggested acupuncture might increase IVF pregnancy rates, but a large review of all of the studies showed acupuncture didn't make much difference. In seven studies of 1,601 women undergoing IVF, 32 percent of those who had acupuncture gave birth, as did 29 percent of the control group. The authors of the review concluded, "There is no evidence of benefit for the use of acupuncture in IVF treatment." I think it's more fair to say that there might be a very small benefit. The most recent study on IVF and acupuncture, too new to be in this analysis, also found no effect. If you're undergoing IVF, with its huge investment, it might be worth it to up your chances 3 percentage points by having acupuncture, particularly if it's something you believe in. If you're doing things the old-fashioned way, it's more of a toss-up whether acupuncture is worth your money and time, especially since there are no studies on acupuncture and natural conception. There also aren't any studies on acupuncture and male fertility, though that may come as a relief to some men. (As one of my guy friends asked, "Where would they stick the needles for that?")

Some women take herbs to boost their fertility. A popular product, Fertility Blend, includes L-arginine and vitex (also known as chasteberry). Among 93 women who had been trying to get pregnant for six months to three years, 26 percent became pregnant after three months on Fertility Blend, compared to 10 percent who received a placebo (control) pill. The women's cycles also improved. A few other studies have shown positive effects for vitex among women with short luteal phases (the time between ovulation and a period). However, most of these studies had small samples and were reported in obscure journals. And there have been no studies at all on fertility and Chinese medicine herbs. There's still so much we don't know about herbs and their effects that it probably pays to be cautious in taking them. Hopefully the coming years will produce more research on how herbs and supplements affect fertility.

It's tempting to think that you might as well take herbs because they can't hurt. But sometimes they can: Some women, especially those with regular cycles, have reported that vitex delayed ovulation and made their cycles worse instead of better (for example, read the reviews of Fertility Blend on drugstore.com). That was true for me. I have very short luteal phases. Since some studies have shown that vitex can lengthen the luteal phase, I started taking it at the recommended dose. But all it did was delay my ovulation, and then during the fifth cycle, I had my shortest luteal phase ever. I stopped taking vitex and my cycles went back to normal. Three months later I was pregnant.

L-arginine, also included in Fertility Blend and recommended in some books, has not been studied among women trying to conceive naturally. In a small study of women undergoing IVF, those who took L-arginine actually produced *fewer* good-quality embryos and were *less* likely to get pregnant. The researchers were surprised by these results, as theoretically L-arginine should help fertility by increasing blood flow. It's hard to say how it would affect natural conception, but these IVF results were enough to convince me not to take it.

Other herbs, like evening primrose oil, are purported to have beneficial effects, but actually don't. (A large review found that evening primrose oil did not alleviate PMS symptoms, though calcium supplements did.) Some women take megadoses of vitamin B6 (more than 100 milligrams) to try to lengthen their luteal phase or improve PMS symptoms, but no studies have examined if that actually works. Plus the National Institutes of Health says that more than 100 milligrams of vitamin B6 a day can potentially be toxic.

Here's another cautionary tale about herbal supplements. The pretty website for the supplement FertiBella, which says it contains many of the same herbs as Fertility Blend, features video success stories from women and claims it has "clinically proven results," with 33 percent more pregnancies among women who took FertiBella versus a placebo. The page includes a link to a PDF that appears to be an article from the *Journal of Obstetrics & Gynecology and Reproductive Biology*. However, neither the article, nor any of the five authors, nor the journal appear in Medline, the comprehensive database of medical journal articles. The journal also does not have a webpage. The article features writing that seems misplaced in a scientific study. It begins, "Medical breakthroughs promise women greater control over their fertility but should they really delay motherhood? More and more women are following the celebrity-led trend of Hollywood A-listers choosing to have babies in their 40s." The PDF of the article cuts off (mid-sentence) after two vague pages and never presents the study results. The lesson here is that the Internet is the new Wild West, and buyer beware. When a treatment says it's clinically proven or published in a medical journal, do your homework and make sure you can trust it.

The overall message: Don't take herbs or other supplements just to try them, because they can sometimes have negative effects on your fertility. If you know someone or read about someone online who took one of these supplements and then got pregnant, remember that it's impossible to tell if the supplement had anything to do with it. And one person is one person, not a study with thousands of people. My advice is to try to get pregnant for six months— just like the women in the Fertility Blend study—before you consider taking herbs or megadoses of vitamins, and then take them only when other fertility tests (semen analysis, HSG to test for open tubes) come back normal, and after checking with your doctor. Your natural fertility might actually serve you better, so don't mess with it until you have to.

DHEA Supplements

In 2003, a 42-year-old single woman named Dwyn Harben arrived at a New York fertility clinic and told doctors she wanted to store embryos for a future pregnancy. Dwyn underwent IVF but produced only three eggs, which is considered a low response. Wanting to improve her chances, Dwyn did some research and came across a study showing promising results for dehydroepiandrosterone (DHEA), an inexpensive hormonal supplement available without a prescription. Dwyn started taking 75 milligrams a day of DHEA, at first without telling her doctors. Four months after starting DHEA, Dwyn produced 6 eggs per cycle, six months later she produced 14, and nine months later she produced 18. She then confessed her DHEA supplementation to her doctors.

Stunned by these results, the doctors suggested DHEA supplements to other patients, especially those who were older or had trouble making enough eggs during IVF treatment. One of them was Melissa, 40, who had suffered infertility for years. Four different infertility clinics told Melissa that she would never have a baby unless she used donor eggs. She then went to the clinic Dwyn had used, the Center for Human Reproduction (CHR), headed by Drs. David Barad and Norbert Gleicher. Initially Melissa had two failed IVF cycles. The doctors suggested she take DHEA, and after five months on the supplement Melissa made an appointment with Dr. Barad because she wasn't feeling well. Dr. Barad did an ultrasound and found the cause for Melissa's nausea and fatigue: She was pregnant—naturally. Her son, Lucas, was born the day before her 41st birthday.

Since then, Drs. Barad and Gleicher have published several papers in top medical journals showing that these women's results were not a fluke. Among several hundred women, DHEA increased the number of embryos produced in IVF cycles, improved pregnancy rates, and decreased the number of abnormal embryos. Best of all, it cut the miscarriage rate in half among women over 35. Only 7 percent of women 35 to 37 years old who took DHEA miscarried, compared to the usual miscarriage rate of 16 percent. Women who took DHEA also produced 38 percent fewer abnormal embryos. And that's from taking a nonprescription supplement that costs about $10 for a month's supply.

Because DHEA is a hormone, some stores put warnings next to the bottles. This made me wonder about the possibility of birth defects. I emailed Dr. Gleicher and he wrote back, "There is no evidence of increased birth defects and no reason to believe that there would be," especially because women stop taking DHEA once they get a positive pregnancy test. In addition, DHEA is naturally found in the body and is higher in women during pregnancy, anyway. ("The placenta is a DHEA factory," he wrote.) And because more embryos were normal among women who took DHEA, there should be a *reduced* risk of chromosomal birth defects such as Down syndrome.

Should you take DHEA? Most of the research is based on IVF, so it's hard to say if it would work for natural conception, though doctors have seen several women, like Melissa, who conceived naturally after taking DHEA. The effectiveness of DHEA is more evident in women over 35 and especially in women over 40. So it might be worth a try if you're over 35 but not if you're younger. If you already know you have high follicle-stimulating hormone (FSH) or diminished ovarian reserve, DHEA might be especially helpful. But because DHEA increases estrogen, much like vitex, it could delay ovulation in a woman with regular cycles. So you might want to try it out for a cycle or two when you're not trying to get pregnant to see how it affects you. Or, like vitex or Fertility Blend, consider taking it only after you've been trying for six months.

The recommended dose for DHEA is 25 milligrams three times a day, and the best effects came after four to five months, so give it at least this long to work. Although current research suggests that DHEA is safe in these amounts, you shouldn't take it for more than a year, and you'll want to stop taking it when you get a positive pregnancy test or if your doctor otherwise tells you to. The research is still in its initial stages, but it's exciting that something—anything—makes a difference for women who thought their only chance for a baby might be donor eggs.

CoQ-10 Supplements

Co-enzyme Q10 is a naturally occurring substance essential for cell formation. The older you are, the less CoQ-10 your body naturally produces. Some exciting emerging research has found that CoQ-10 supplements are effective in treating diseases from high blood pressure to diabetes, with no side effects or adverse events. Because ovulation involves a long process of cell development, adequate levels of CoQ-10 are essential for fertility. Unfortunately, no one has yet studied the effect of CoQ-10 on human fertility. One study found that older female mice that ate CoQ-10 supplements produced better eggs. (Mice are considered old at a year, which makes me feel lucky to be human.) If you're older than 35, CoQ-10 might be worth a try, at a dose of 100 milligrams a day.

Stress

"Just relax and you'll get pregnant." This is some of the most common advice you'll hear about fertility. But is it right? Do we have to de-stress and even stop worrying about our fertility to have a child?

Probably not. Your body adjusts to your level of normal day-to-day stress. Unusual events—like moving, breaking a bone, or traveling for long periods—can affect your cycle, usually by delaying ovulation. Simple worry about getting pregnant is unlikely to decrease your fertility. Neither is "trying too hard" by predicting your ovulation, getting ready to get pregnant, or eating well. You've probably heard the stories about women who finally got pregnant when they adopted a child or otherwise "stopped trying," but one doesn't cause the other. (Research doesn't show any link—stories are just stories. Psychologists call this an *illusory correlation.*) In fact, "trying too hard" by knowing your cycle is *more* likely to lead to a quick conception.

Most studies show that anxiety and mild to moderate stress do not affect fertility, even during fertility treatment. Alice Domar, a psychologist well known for her studies on how psychological therapy can help infertile women get pregnant, reported that women with moderate levels of anxiety were actually *more* likely to conceive with IVF. A 2011 analysis of 14 studies found no differences in IVF pregnancy rates among women who were stressed versus not. Toni Weschler, the author of *Taking Charge of Your Fertility*, writes that stress delays ovulation but doesn't otherwise harm fertility when trying to conceive naturally. So anxiety is nothing to get anxious about unless it's debilitating.

Unfortunately, many gynecologists have not gotten this message. Some doctors tell their patients just to "have fun" or "have lots of sex" because they believe that predicting ovulation and "obsessing" about getting pregnant can harm fertility. That's just not true. Taking a laid-back approach can certainly work, but predicting your ovulation will help you get pregnant faster—and then you can stop stressing about getting pregnant. One woman posted on a message board that at her preconception appointment the doctor "told me not to chart, not to read anything, and especially not to go on the Internet." (Why? Because ignorance causes pregnancy?) The woman continued, "I'm glad I didn't listen to her because I knew what I needed to do to increase my chances. I think I would have driven myself crazy *not* knowing what my body was doing."

Jackie, an anthropology professor, is a perfect example

of how short-term stress doesn't necessarily lower fertility. Jackie tried to get pregnant on her own for two years. She then took Clomid for a few cycles and tried intrauterine insemination (IUI), but neither worked. Right before her second IUI, her department chair told her that she might not get tenure. She went for the IUI anyway, and her doctor knew right away that Jackie was stressed out because the regular catheter wouldn't go in and he had to use a more flexible one. Jackie wondered how she could possibly get pregnant less than an hour after the worst meeting of her life, but she did—with twins! (And she got tenure after all.)

Depression, however, *does* negatively affect fertility. Most studies, again on IVF patients, find that depressed women are less than half as likely to get pregnant as those who aren't depressed. What's the difference between stress and depression? If you're worried, or obsessed, or keyed up, that's stress. If you're sad, crying all the time, or lethargic for more than two weeks, that's depression. (Feeling sad for a few days after getting your period doesn't count—it has to go on longer than that.) If you are depressed or think you might be, consider starting therapy—for your own mental health, not just for fertility. Most psychologists, including Dr. Domar, recommend a program that uses cognitive-behavioral therapy and progressive relaxation techniques. (For more, see *Feeling Good* or *The Relaxation Response*.) Therapy is probably a better choice than antidepressant medications, some of which shouldn't be used during pregnancy. If you're already taking an antidepressant or considering doing so, you should talk to your doctor about your options.

I'll say more about the psychological aspects of getting pregnant in Chapter 7 and throughout the book, because trying to get pregnant can be so stressful. Even if the stress doesn't affect your fertility, it's still no fun to feel anxious all of the time. Many people assume that trying to get pregnant is pure fun and that stress and/or depression doesn't set in until infertility treatment begins. However, I've met women who were anxious about their fertility before they even started trying and even more who worried about never getting pregnant after their first or second cycle wasn't successful. Having children is such an important life goal, yet it's not under our control. If you are already prone to anxiety, the inherent stress of trying to get pregnant can make it worse. The good news is that a low or even moderate level of anxiety and obsessiveness is unlikely to harm your fertility.

What if you work long hours and have a stressful job? If that means you don't sleep enough, eat unhealthy food, and live on caffeine and alcohol, then yes, you might have more trouble getting pregnant. But in that case it's the caffeine, alcohol, and bad food—not the stress—that are having negative effects. Some women get the idea that they won't be able to get pregnant unless they are relaxing all the time, and that's just not true. As with most things, a middle ground is probably the best place to be—finding a lifestyle that keeps you busy and engaged in life, but not so busy that you're going crazy.

One way to find that balance is by setting aside enough time for sleep and relaxation. To sleep well, it's important to use your bed only for sleep and baby-making—no reading or watching TV in bed, and especially no working in bed. That way, you will learn to associate your bed with relaxation and rest. Turn off your cell phone before you go to bed and leave it in another room. Try to have at least an hour to relax before you go to sleep—read a book, take a bath, or watch TV. Doing any of these in the dark or with just a little reading light is especially effective, as the dark lets your brain know that it's almost bedtime. This means no working right before bed, because unless you're completely exhausted, you're not going to be able to instantly turn your brain off and go to sleep.

Spreading the News—or Not

Once you've decided to start trying to get pregnant, you might feel an immediate urge to tell everyone. Squash it. You don't want to announce, "We're trying!" to too many people, because then the same number of people will be asking you, "Are you pregnant yet?" a month later. You'll probably be tempted to tell your mother, but hold off on that for a few months. If you get pregnant right away, you can just share the happy news with your mom, and if you don't, you can cry on her shoulder. Moms can be a great source of support, but sometimes they can make you feel more anxious or give you outdated advice. What about telling your dad? Unless you have a very unusual father, don't go there. As much as they love us, dads live by a simple rule when it comes to the sex lives of their daughters: They don't want to know.

You'll probably end up telling your closest girlfriends, especially if they've already tried to conceive. Even if they haven't, you should be able to count on them for emotional support. Girlfriends are also partners in crime for obsessing over your fertility signs (see Chapter 3). Try not to overwhelm your husband with details about your cycles—the less he has to know, the happier you will both be. (In Chapter 4, I'll say more about seduction methods more pleasant than yelling, "I'm ovulating! Get in here!")

Should you join an online discussion group of other women who are trying to conceive? Some women love them, but others find it strange to disclose details about cervical mucus to strangers. There's more about online message boards in Chapter 7. If you've never been on a trying-to-conceive message board, be aware that they love acronyms almost as much as the military does. (I've included a cheat sheet in Appendix B.) It leads to sentences like, "I got a BFP on my OPK, so me and my DH BD'd. Now in the 2WW. Praying for no AF!" (Translation: "I got a positive on an ovulation predictor, so my husband and I had sex. I'm now in the two-week wait [after ovulation, before testing]. Praying I don't get my period.") Message boards sound a lot like Robin Williams' parody of army-speak in the movie *Good Morning Vietnam*: "Seeing how the VP is such a VIP, shouldn't we keep the PC on the QT, because if it leaks to the VC, you could end up an MIA, and then we'd all be put on KP." Just try not to go too far to the military side in your TTC quest or you'll end up barking orders at your husband: "Operation ovulation has commenced! All soldiers at attention! Get ready for imminent insertion!"

Planning When to Get Pregnant, and How Long It Might Take

If we Impatient Women waited until the perfect time to get pregnant, with nothing pressing on our schedules, we'd end up like the woman in the cartoon who says, "I can't believe I forgot to have children!" But many of us do have good and bad times during the year for our careers, or travel plans, or friends' weddings that we don't want to be fat or barfing for. Which of these, if any, to make a priority is a personal choice. One possibility is to identify a good time to start trying and plan for it, realizing that you want to allow at least a three- to four-month window to get pregnant.

When planning your pregnancy, you'll probably think first about when you will deliver: Is it a good time to take maternity leave? A good time to stay at home and not travel? Keep in mind that your baby might arrive a week, a month, or even two months early. But don't just think about your due date. Also consider your commitments and plans during the months right after you start trying, when you might be in your first trimester and feeling really awful. The symptoms are likely to kick in when you're about six weeks pregnant. You've probably heard about the nausea that characterizes early pregnancy. Most women are also very tired and unenergetic. Unfortunately the fatigue doesn't go away even if you sleep for 9 or 10 hours a night (which you will).

Early pregnancy can feel like having a bad flu for several months. Apparently this fatigue is partially caused by your uterus building the placenta that will support your baby. (When I learned that, I immediately blurted that after the birth I was going to pummel the crap out of that stupid placenta. Maybe I should have done that and filmed it—it might have gone viral on YouTube.) It's safe to travel in your first trimester, but you will need to eat very frequently (that helps with the nausea) and sleep just as much or more as you do at home. You won't be able to take most medications such as sleeping pills. If you have allergies, try to have your first trimester (and ideally the entire pregnancy) fall outside of your usual allergy season. If that's not possible, talk to your doctor about safe options for allergy relief during pregnancy.

Of course, at some point all of these considerations have to get kicked down the priority list and you just have to make do. I ended up traveling for work, sometimes cross-country, several times a month during my first trimester with our second child. I tried to get as much rest as I could and packed as much food as I could. It was tough, but I did it. If I could have pinpointed when I'd be pregnant, that wouldn't have been my choice, but after a few months of trying and an early miscarriage, I decided I didn't care anymore and that a healthy baby was more important. And she was.

If you already have one or more young children and you're thinking about getting pregnant again, you're probably giving a lot of thought to child spacing. A few studies have shown it's healthier to space pregnancies at least 18 months apart (so at least 18 months between delivering one child and getting pregnant with the next, which would put the children at least 2 years and 3 months apart). This results in fewer complications such as low birth weight, probably because the woman's body has had enough time to recover and build up her nutritional stores. It also gives you time to enjoy each of your children before another comes on the scene—or you're pregnant and barely capable of lying on the couch. Our first child, then 2, watched an appalling amount of television when I was pregnant with our second (the theme music from her favorite show still makes me vaguely nauseous). One woman told me, "As soon as you're pregnant, your focus shifts to the next one. So give it time." Of course, many older IWs who want two or more children will feel they don't have the luxury of that much time. If that's your situation, consider compromising by waiting until your current baby is at least a year old. You'll be much more recovered than you were at six months or even nine months, your baby will be a somewhat more independent toddler, and it's more likely that your cycles will have returned to normal after nursing.

Choose your first month of trying very carefully. Don't automatically assume it will take six months to get pregnant. A lot of books and websites say that the chances of pregnancy each cycle are only 15 percent to 25 percent if you're younger than 35 and 5 percent to 10 percent if you're older. Many also say that it takes a 30-year-old woman an average of seven months to get pregnant. I have no idea where these statistics come from, because according to the published research, they're wrong. One study found that women in their late 20s or early 30s who had sex at least twice a week got pregnant, on average, within three months. For those 35 to 39, the average was four months. Another found that women in their late 20s or early 30s who had sex two days before ovulation—and *only* on that cycle day—got pregnant 35 percent of the time. The odds are even higher if you can predict your ovulation using the techniques I'll reveal in

Chapter 3. Between 67 percent and 76 percent of women under 35 who were aware of their fertile time conceived in the *first month*. If you use the methods of fertility awareness I describe in this book, you have a good chance of getting pregnant the very first time you try. So make sure your first cycle isn't too early for what you're planning. But also realize that you might not get lucky the first time, and that doesn't mean anything is wrong. (Plus your husband will be thrilled to keep trying a little longer.)

If you've already been trying for longer than three months, *please* don't panic. It's very possible you're just timing things wrong. Even if you've been using ovulation predictor kits, a fertility monitor, or charting, your timing can still be off. Chapter 4 tells you how to pinpoint the best time to have sex—which is not when many sources say it is. It's also possible you just haven't hit the right month yet. Even the study finding 75 percent of women getting pregnant right away stated that it took the rest anywhere from two to seven months even when they were timing things exactly right.

If you're anxious about the process, though, you are far from alone. Anne, 34, says, "I thought we would get pregnant the second we looked at each other without protection. My mom and sister both got pregnant once they went off birth control." But that didn't happen. "The sense of urgency kicked in when we were still trying at month 6. At month 10, I began to panic!" Fortunately, Anne got pregnant soon afterward and had a healthy baby boy. One wise young woman I know took a more philosophical approach. "If it works, it works; and if there's a problem, there are many different ways to have a baby," she wrote. If only we could all be that calm.

CHAPTER 2

Supplements, Exercise, and the SOS Diet

So much has been written about food and diets that it's easy to get impatient with all of the advice. There's also lots of discussion about weight, from weighing too little to weighing too much, with diet and exercise plans going in and out of fashion.

The research on fertility and weight is fairly clear. Women who weigh too much and those who weigh too little take longer to get pregnant—twice as long for those who are seriously overweight and four times as long for underweight women. Maximum fertility occurs at a body mass index (BMI) between 20 and 24. (You can find your BMI by entering your weight and height into an online calculator.)

For fertility, being underweight is a bigger problem than being overweight. Women who don't have enough body fat may stop getting periods, which means they're not ovulating. If you are very thin (with a BMI of 19 or below), you might need to gain some weight and scale back your exercise to increase your chances of getting pregnant, especially if your cycles are irregular or absent. The good news is your fertility will likely return once your BMI is 20 or higher. It might feel strange to eat more and exercise less—you've probably always prided yourself on your healthy lifestyle—but women need a little body fat to get pregnant. The fat doesn't have to come from ice cream or chips. Try healthy fat sources like nuts, salmon, seeds, and avocados. If you don't gain weight fast enough on those foods, some studies suggest that whole milk has fertility benefits.

If you're overweight (with a BMI of 25 or higher), losing weight may benefit your fertility. Sometimes it can make all the difference. One episode of *I Didn't Know I Was Pregnant* featured Susan and her husband, who had given up on having a baby after trying for more than a decade. At 40, Susan had gastric bypass surgery and lost 90 pounds. She felt some strange sensations in her abdomen on and off throughout the summer and fall, and then, at a Halloween party, found herself doubled over with pain. When she got to the hospital, she was told she was pregnant—and in labor. A few hours later she delivered the daughter she never thought she'd have. More than likely, the weight loss from the surgery made her fertile.

Unless you are seriously overweight, though, chances are you don't need surgery—just a better diet and an exercise plan. Even if you are a normal weight, eating healthier can help. The eating plan that follows can boost fertility, and it might help you lose weight as well.

What to Put in Your Mouth

No, not that—you can't get pregnant that way (no matter what your husband says)! I'm talking about what you eat and the vitamins and supplements you take.

Most important: Start taking a prenatal vitamin about two months before you start trying to get pregnant so that the nutrients have enough time to build up in your body before the crucial first trimester. Most prenatal vitamins don't include enough calcium, so take a separate calcium supplement with vitamin D, ideally after a low-calcium meal. (Your body can absorb only so much calcium at one time and absorbs it better after a meal.) A calcium supplement can be a pill or—my personal chocoholic favorite—a chocolate- or caramel-flavored chew. Calcium keeps you strong. If your baby doesn't get enough calcium when you're pregnant, it takes calcium from your bones (the little vampire!) and you're more likely to get osteoporosis. Some studies have found that calcium helps with PMS symptoms. And some very exciting emerging research finds that vitamin D promotes good health in everything from fertility to cancer prevention. Several studies have found that women taking prenatal vitamins, especially folate and vitamin B6, are more likely to get pregnant quickly. New research also suggests that taking prenatal vitamins before conception can lower the risk of autism.

When you comparison shop for prenatal vitamins, don't assume that the cheaper ones are bad. Most expensive prenatal vitamins have blends of antioxidants and other stuff that's nice but not essential. Just make sure the vitamin has enough folic acid (sometimes called folate; at least 800 micrograms), enough iron (about 25 milligrams), and enough vitamin B6 (about 10 milligrams). Folic acid, especially when taken before conception and early in pregnancy, greatly reduces the chance of having a baby with a neural tube defect (like anencephaly, when the baby is born with a tiny brain and only lives a few hours, or spina bifida, an exposed spine). If you're uncertain about taking supplements because you already have a healthy diet, keep in mind that it's very hard to get enough folic acid and iron from food alone, and the studies on folic acid suggest that supplements are more effective at preventing birth defects than natural folate.

Also consider taking an omega-3 supplement of fish oil (sometimes labeled DHA or EPA). One study of women undergoing IVF found that those with higher omega-3 levels produced better embryos. Some studies (though not all) have found that women who consume more omega-3 fatty acids during pregnancy have smarter babies, possibly because omega-3 is necessary for brain development. The benefits of omega-3 go beyond fertility: People who get enough omega-3 fatty acids are less likely to get heart disease or to become depressed. Fish oil supplements are especially important if you never eat fish. If you're a vegetarian and don't want to take fish oil, you can consider flaxseed oil. However, flaxseed oil takes much longer to convert to omega-3 in your body, so you'll want to research this option further.

The Benefits of Eating Healthy
Before You Get Pregnant

Even if you take vitamins and supplements, you still have to eat nutritious food, beginning a few months before you start trying to get pregnant. You might be asking, "Do I really have to worry about this now? Can't I eat healthy once I get pregnant?" You can try, but you might spend most of your first trimester eating total junk like white bread and pizza. It's more of a mandate than a craving; to keep from feeling hungry and nauseous (these two are the same thing in early pregnancy), you have to eat all the time, and starchy carbs are most likely to make you feel full and thus less likely to make you feel like tossing up your carbs. Supposedly, Gwyneth Paltrow hadn't eaten white bread in three years before she got pregnant with her first child, but then she said, "It was like, 'Pass the biscuits.'" During my first trimesters, even the thought of eating anything green made me want to hurl. I subsisted on pizza, sandwiches, bread, bread, and more bread. My favorite was the frozen Tandoori Naan from Trader Joe's, which cooks in three minutes flat and fills the kitchen with the smell of, you guessed it, bread. In my third pregnancy I found a whole-wheat Tandoori at Whole Foods, which was even better.

So it's up to your prepregnant self to eat healthy, because your postpregnant self probably won't, at least not in the first three months. It takes time for nutrients to build up in your body—you are what you ate two or three months ago. So when you get pregnant, your baby will be snacking off everything you ate *before* you got pregnant. This advice is based on another amazing fact: Your baby's heart, brain, spinal cord, and other major organs will be almost completely formed just 8 weeks after conception. That's why it's a good idea to improve your diet, take prenatal vitamins and supplements, and stop eating high-mercury fish a few months *before* you start trying. Some doctors call this the "Twelve-Month Pregnancy," which is, admittedly, a scary thought. Fortunately, the first three months—those before you get pregnant—mostly involve eating good food and having sex, so it's not so bad.

If you've had a hard time motivating yourself to eat healthy before, thinking about having a healthy baby might be the inspiration you need. Don't get overly stressed or scared about any of this—women are under enough pressure about food already. Make some positive changes, but don't think you have to be perfect.

I have an enormous sweet tooth and don't like most vegetables. Before I got pregnant the first time, I read the nutrition books that stressed the importance of eating green leafy vegetables, so I tried to eat salads for lunch. After a few weeks, I was hungry and miserable. I realized things weren't working when the only way I could get down the spinach and romaine was by cramming a handful into my mouth, chewing as quickly as possible, and washing it down with juice. Pretty dumb. So I don't buy salad bags anymore. I eat raw spinach on sandwiches and put romaine lettuce on turkey burgers and tacos, and I get the rest of my green veggies from broccoli and bok choy, which I like marginally better. I also eat veggies first, when I'm the most hungry. You'll find your own way of working in the foods you should eat but don't want to. The main thing is to find some compromise between eating what you want (fries and a cupcake) and what you should (healthy food). If you like fries, for example, try baked sweet potato fries or sliced potatoes, but treat them as the starch for your dinner, not the vegetable.

So what should you eat? It spells SOS: spinach, olives, and salmon (each of these is a stand-in for a larger group of healthy foods). What shouldn't you eat? Another S: Stuff (or another s-word) that's bad for you—more on that later.

Will a Healthy Diet Help You Get Pregnant?

The quick answer to this question is maybe. The best-known series of studies, summarized in the book *The Fertility Diet*, found dietary changes were effective only for preventing ovulatory infertility, such as lack of ovulation and hormonal imbalances. Because the women in the studies ate what they wanted, the researchers can't say that diet caused fertility, because an outside factor could have caused both. (Perhaps, for example, women with higher incomes were more likely to eat in a certain way and more likely to get pregnant, so maybe it wasn't diet that caused higher fertility but better resources. Keep this caveat in mind for all of the studies about fertility and diet.) It's also possible that the results were driven primarily by women with polycystic ovarian syndrome (a disorder that affects ovulation) and might not apply to women without this disorder. Even so, other studies have started to confirm that diet can affect fertility, and they are fairly consistent in their findings. The SOS diet, an IW exclusive, brings together all of these research findings in an easy-to-remember acronym.

Let's start with the first S in SOS: spinach. The good news is you don't necessarily have to eat spinach, just healthy food in general: fruits, vegetables, and whole grains. Use spinach as a cue to remember all of this healthy stuff. The studies in *The Fertility Diet* found that women who ate these types of healthy foods were 92 percent less likely to suffer from ovulatory infertility than those who ate processed foods like pastries, white bread, pizza, sugary drinks, potatoes, and white pasta. They also found better fertility among those who ate vegetarian sources of protein such as beans, nuts, and soy instead of animal meats. These findings bring to mind the succinct advice of author Michael Pollan: "Eat food. Not too much. Mostly plants." That means brown rice, whole-wheat bread, beans, fruits, vegetables, whole-wheat pasta, tofu, lentils, and nuts.

These suggestions reminded me of the unappetizing plates of black beans and vegetables that vegetarian friends of mine used to eat in the university dining hall (at which I would usually glance briefly while I was stuffing my face with pizza). Although I've never been significantly overweight, I was a very slow convert to any type of health food. For one thing, most nutrition books presume that you actually know how to cook. Well into my 20s, I was convinced that nonmicrowavable food was not worth the trouble unless it was, say, cookies, and even then I preferred the raw dough straight out of the package. (Is there a meeting for that?) Nutrition books also featured long lists of weird junk I couldn't imagine eating. (What is blackstrap molasses, anyway? It sounds sticky. And how about some Swiss chard for dinner? Yum.) Healthy food sounded like too much trouble, too much money, and too weird to a Midwesterner like me who grew up eating Spaghetti-Os and Jell-O. To start eating healthy, I had to improvise. Slowly, I found out that eating healthy doesn't have to involve exotic products, time-consuming cooking, or expensive food. (The standard nickname for Whole Foods is "Whole Paycheck," and if you've shopped there you know why.)

Mostly, I read labels. I still eat cereal with skim milk for breakfast, but I only buy cereal with more than 4 grams of fiber per serving (an indicator of whole grains). High-fiber cereal and oatmeal, as it turns out, are some of the best sources of fiber and very easy to prepare. I even tried steel-cut oats, which are a true whole grain, though I usually stick with instant oatmeal (which are rolled oats—not a completely whole grain, but a lot closer than Coco Puffs). I often have microwave dinners for lunch, but I choose ones with whole grains, fiber, vegetables, and lean protein. Especially between meals, I drink water instead of soda or juice. (This one change alone helped me lose 10 pounds during my early thirties.)

I started making dinners that always included a vegetable and searched for better starches like brown rice and barley. Although whole-wheat bread, cereal, and pasta are much better for you than refined grains like white bread, they are still not a completely whole grain like wild rice or quinoa (pronounced keen-wa, believe it or not). So I cut back on bread and pasta, even the whole-wheat versions. I found a $10 rice cooker that cooked all kinds of raw whole grains perfectly and got some 90-second microwavable rice packets (often from Trader Joe's or Whole Foods) that had a mix of whole grains with lots of fiber. I'm not a vegetarian (the not liking vegetables or beans ruled that out), so the protein portion is fish or poultry, either grilled or baked. I hate chopping vegetables, so I buy the packets of pre-chopped veggies. Although I now use appliances other than the microwave, I usually spend no more than 15 minutes cooking. And I still eat pizza, but intersperse it with more healthy fare. For snacks, I often eat nuts like cashews and fresh fruit like strawberries.

My diet is not perfect, but I now eat more healthy food that doesn't break the bank, tastes pretty good, and doesn't try my very limited patience for cooking. My basic point: If a pizza-loving, chocolate-addicted, noncooking, bean-hating person like me can eat healthy, so can you. Improve your diet as much as you can and you'll see results.

In the end, I even tried some of the funky stuff mentioned in the nutrition books. I thought quinoa sounded like something only a wacko foodie would eat, but it turns out you can make it in a microwave or a rice cooker with virtually no effort, and it's delicious. It also has more protein and fiber than almost any other grain. I never expected to like bok choy, but it's not bad when you cook the leaves in a skillet with olive oil, salt, and garlic powder. My 4-year-old eats bok choy and says it's her favorite, which is probably a sign of the apocalypse. The specter of onrushing gloom usually recedes when she finishes the bok choy and says, "Can I have dessert now?"—reassuring proof that she was not switched at the hospital.

The second part of the SOS plan is olives, which is a memory cue for a Mediterranean diet with foods such as olive oil, fish, vegetables, and legumes (like beans, peas, or peanuts). In a study of 161 women undergoing IVF, those who followed a Mediterranean diet were 40 percent more likely to get pregnant. Of course, olive oil is still a refined oil, so it's best used sparingly, usually as a substitute for butter or another vegetable oil. And if you can eat the actual olive instead, that's even better. The authors of this study speculate that the Mediterranean diet may increase fertility because it boosts blood levels of folate and vitamin B6.

Though I can't claim to have a completely Mediterranean diet, I've tried to follow a few of its principles, like eating more fish and vegetables. I use olive oil for cooking instead of butter, and I even use it for making cookies and cakes when the box calls for vegetable oil. The finished product tastes the same and it's better for you. (Not as good as avoiding cookies and cake in the first place, but who are we kidding?)

To Fish or Not to Fish?

You've probably heard lots of confusing things about whether you should eat fish. Some fish contain mercury, and if you eat too much of these fish—even before you get pregnant—the mercury could have adverse effects on your baby. But fish is a great source of lean protein and is by far the best source for omega-3 fatty acids, which are essential for a baby's brain development. *The Fertility Diet* studies found that fish is better for fertility than poultry or red meat. So what gives—should you eat fish or not?

The quick answer: Yes, but only some types. Only some fish have high levels of mercury, and only some have high levels of omega-3s. Fortunately, one common fish has the right combination of low mercury and high omega-3s: salmon. So the last S in SOS is salmon. Trout, arctic char, herring, whitefish, and oysters are also low in mercury and high in omega-3s, but salmon often is the easiest to find.

There's a lot of conflicting information about salmon and PCB (polychlorinated biphenyl) contamination: Some studies find higher levels in farmed salmon and others in wild, and most suggest that the salmon available in the United States is relatively low in PCBs. One study looked specifically at PCB levels in women's blood and found no link to fertility. I can't give you a definitive answer about how much you should worry about PCBs, though I can say that the evidence linking fish with smarter babies outweighs the negative evidence on PCBs in salmon. You can also consider finding a happy medium for salmon consumption, perhaps no more than twice a week—enough to get the beneficial omega-3s but not overdo it in case of any contamination.

Other fish with at least moderate amounts of omega-3s include halibut, pollock (often found in breaded fish), flounder, sea bass, and sole. Even seafood with fewer omega-3s, like mahi mahi, shrimp, scallops, and cod, are great sources of lean protein. Avoid very high-mercury fish like shark, swordfish, king mackerel, and tilefish. Find a website that lists the average mercury content for each type of fish. If you see a fish you'd like to try (say, at a restaurant), ask how big the fish is; bigger fish usually have more mercury contamination than smaller fish. Fish with moderate levels of mercury include halibut, mahi mahi, and any kind of tuna, including canned. Have no more than three moderate-mercury fish servings a month, especially right before you start trying to get pregnant and during the first trimester. Put all of these rules into place at least three months *before* you start trying, because mercury takes months to leave your body, and the developing baby is the most vulnerable in the first trimester. Some seafood has virtually no mercury, so you can eat as much as you'd like; these include salmon, tilapia, flounder, clams, herring, pollock, shrimp, scallops, and catfish.

The Food and Drug Administration's official statement on mercury gives an upper limit of 12 ounces for fish consumption a week, but it doesn't specify what type of fish (except not to eat shark, swordfish, king mackerel, or tilefish). That's really silly, because you can gorge yourself on 24 ounces of salmon in a week and get very little mercury exposure, but if you eat 12 ounces of tuna, even canned tuna, every week, that's too much. Two to three servings of tuna or four servings of halibut add up to just as much mercury exposure as one serving of swordfish, one of the fish on the "no" list. That doesn't mean you should never have tuna or halibut—just that you should limit your intake. You have to do the math to really understand how much mercury exposure you're getting.

What if you hate fish? Consider giving it another try. Yes, I know I sound like a mother trying to get her 4-year-old to eat (probably because I am a mother with a 4-year-old). For years I thought I hated salmon because I'd had it once at a college function—it was dry and covered in a mysterious sauce. When I tried it again years later, I really liked it—and that was when I put it on a Foreman grill for a few minutes. With some soy or teriyaki sauce, it's even better. There are so many different types of fish that almost everyone will like at least one of them. Fish is also really easy to make, especially if your husband likes to grill. (The easiest cooking is that done by someone else!) Or try it first at a restaurant where they specialize in fish—you'll realize quickly just how good it can taste, and you'll then be more willing to try it again.

Organic Food and Dairy: Let the Debate Begin

Do you need to eat organic food when you're trying to get pregnant? That's a matter of heated debate. Organic food is expensive, often costing twice as much as conventionally grown food. It's also not available everywhere, especially if you're outside a big city (or even if you're inside—the closest Whole Foods to my house is a 30-minute drive even though I live in a major metropolitan area in California). Many books and websites recommend organic food for fertility even though no study has shown that those who eat organic are more fertile. When I searched for "organic food" and "fertility" in the comprehensive medical journal database Medline, there were no articles—not a single study.

Whether you're an organic food advocate or not, keep an open mind and try to evaluate what you hear from a scientific point of view. So far, the debate has generated reams of commentary but very little data. When conventional food advocates say there is little evidence that pesticides are harmful, it doesn't mean that pesticide exposure is safe—just that we don't know. And when studies do find a link, like one finding that kids who ate conventionally grown produce (versus organic) were more likely to have attention deficit hyperactivity disorder (ADHD), remember that isn't proof that one caused the other, because ADHD and diet could be caused by something else (like income level or ethnic group.) In addition, organic food has less pesticide residue, but it may have more contamination from manure (otherwise known as animal poop). Food is big business, and the debate over these issues is not likely to die down anytime soon. Right now, we don't know enough to say that eating organic is always better.

One way to split the difference is to buy organic versions of the "dirty dozen" (in terms of pesticide residue) of fruits and vegetables (including strawberries, peaches, celery, pears, and apples) and stick with the cheaper conventional versions of milk, grains, and poultry. Buying local produce may be more important than buying organic, because it's more likely to be fresh and thus more nutritious and better tasting. If you already eat organic, stay with it as long as you are also eating a healthy diet. Just remember that not all organic food is healthy. You can buy organic cheese puffs, organic sugary cereal, and organic cookies, but that doesn't mean you should. Organic evaporated cane juice is still sugar!

What about dairy? A lot of fertility books advise against

eating dairy, but *The Fertility Diet* research studies found that full-fat dairy (such as whole milk and ice cream) actually improved fertility, lowering the risk of ovulation problems. The researchers aren't sure exactly why. They speculate that the skimming process for making low-fat and fat-free milk might also remove other beneficial substances. Given that full-fat dairy adds a lot of saturated fat and calories, this is a tough choice to make. You could consider switching to full-fat for a few months while trying to get pregnant, but only if your weight is already under control.

One good dairy choice is yogurt. Even people who have trouble with other dairy foods can often eat yogurt, and it has important probiotics. Unfortunately, most yogurt is sweetened with loads of refined sugar, and plain yogurt tastes awful (to me—if you like it, more power to you). If you can find yogurt with fruit on the bottom, buy that and eat just the yogurt on top—there's enough flavor for it to taste good, but you can leave most of the sugar behind. Or buy plain yogurt and mix in fruit baby food (Gerber's Banana and Mixed Berries is my favorite, sweet enough to cut the bitterness of plain yogurt). Baby food has no artificial sugar added, so you're sweetening your yogurt with puréed fruit only. I don't know why the yogurt makers don't do this themselves.

If you don't do well with dairy, there are lots of other ways to get enough calcium. The easiest is a calcium supplement. Leafy greens like bok choy, collard greens, and kale have a surprising amount of calcium. Soy milk and rice milk are often fortified with calcium, and you can also buy calcium-fortified orange juice.

What Not to Eat

Two food types increase the risk of ovulatory infertility: sweetened carbonated beverages (like soda, which you already know is bad for you) and trans fat (also known as partially hydrogenated oils, or, as I like to call them, partially hydrogenated evil). One study found that women with high blood levels of trans fats were 80 to 90 percent less likely to get pregnant during IVF.

Fortunately, trans fat's long crime spree through the American diet has mostly been halted; the cookies, baked goods, and other foods that used to contain trans fat have mostly been modified to banish the substance. Most evil oils are safely in bad food jail.

But not all. I'll save you some time scrutinizing food labels and tell you the one food that still employs significant amounts of felon trans fat: frosting. I say that with considerable regret, because I think frosting is the best food on the planet. I regularly eat the top of a cupcake—the frosting and about a fourth of the cake—and leave the rest of the cake orphaned on the plate. Cake is merely a frosting delivery mechanism. Unfortunately, the labels on tubs of cake frosting—which I read while I eat it straight out of the can with a spoon—reveal several grams of trans fat. I've found a few ready-made cakes that are sans trans fat (a good one is made by Just Dessert), but other trans-fat-free frosting I've tried has the consistency of wallpaper paste. If you're trying to get pregnant or will in the next three months, frosting moderation is probably in order.

Some margarine and peanut butter still contain trans fat,

so read labels carefully. Where possible, use real butter—or, even better, olive oil. Trans fat also lurks in other foods but doesn't always show up in the Nutrition Facts label. Food labels list grams of trans fat (it's found right under the general heading for fat content that comes first on the label). But if there's less than 0.5 grams of trans fat per serving, the label can still say 0 grams. So if you eat more than one serving—and sometimes servings can be unrealistically small—you could end up ingesting several grams of trans fat. (*The Fertility Diet* research found negative effects at the level of 4 grams of trans fat a day.) If you're eating several servings of a food, read the ingredient label for hidden trans fat. If you see partially hydrogenated oil, the food item has fugitive trans fat in it. Reading ingredients is also a good idea for food that doesn't come with a Nutrition Facts label but does have an ingredient list, like bakery cakes (hmmm, and cupcakes . . . I need to go to the store now).

Exercise

How much should you exercise when you're trying to get pregnant? Welcome to yet another topic that's generated lots of controversy. Women who exercise a lot—really, really a lot, like professional athletes and marathon runners—often have impaired fertility. Sometimes they stop getting periods entirely or have a short luteal phase (the time between ovulation and your period). But what about hitting the gym on a regular basis? That can increase your fertility, partially because it helps you keep your weight down.

One study found that women who engaged in "vigorous" exercise five or more hours a week were 40 percent less likely to experience ovulatory infertility; two to five hours per week lowered the risk 13 percent. Even when weight was taken out of the equation, exercise benefited fertility, with 33 percent less ovulatory infertility among those exercising vigorously five or more hours a week. So what does "vigorous" mean? A few examples: walking 5 miles an hour or faster; jogging or running; bicycling more than 10 miles per hour or going uphill; using a stair climber machine at a fast pace; swimming laps; circuit weight training; playing soccer. (One list I found had fun entries like "square dancing—energetically" and "clogging." Does that refer to shoes or beating? Or beating with shoes? It also listed "rugby," which you probably don't want to indulge in when you're trying to conceive.) The study found that "moderate"-intensity exercise (slower walking or bicycling, nonlap swimming, playing softball, gardening, housework) didn't impact fertility. Keep in mind, though, that this study only looked at infertility due to ovulatory issues—just like the one with food. Nevertheless, exercise might benefit you. It's a great way to lose weight if you need to and an excellent mood booster. And you might end up exercising by chasing around a couple of kids.

CHAPTER 3

Not the Kind of Egg That Comes in a Carton: How to Figure Out When You Are Ovulating

Ah, high school—raging hormones, trying to learn algebra, and suffering through crushes. It was also probably the last time you took a class on reproduction—and, if your crush was in your health class, you probably didn't learn much. I spent most of freshman year health thinking about my crush even though he wasn't in the class. (He eventually married the prom queen, so I missed out on all that information for nothing!)

The main message of most high school health classes is that you can get pregnant anytime—even if he pulls out or if he just ejaculates near you. Apparently sperm can crawl across the backseats of cars. In other words, getting pregnant is easy—way too easy.

But when you're no longer a teenager and actually *want* to get pregnant, somehow it's not so easy. If you don't have sex on the days right before you ovulate (release an egg), you're very unlikely to get pregnant. Sperm live for 2 to 5 days, the little rascals—but the egg only lives about 12 hours on average. So we Impatient Women need to know when we ovulate and we need to know in advance.

There's a common myth that women always ovulate on day 14. Not true. First, most women don't have 28-day cycles, especially not every single month. The pill creates a 28-day cycle, but a natural cycle anywhere from 21 to 35 days is considered normal. Ovulation can happen from as early as 7 days after you get your period to 40 or more days afterward. You might also have heard that women ovulate 14 days before their period. That's not true, either. The time between ovulation and your period (called the luteal phase) can vary from 7 days to 19 days; 14 days is the most common, but it's far from the only option. From one cycle to another, an individual woman's luteal phase is usually about the same length, varying by only a day or so, but your usual length could be shorter or longer than the average of 14 days. So having sex a few times around what you think is the middle of your cycle might not cut it.

If you're merely a Semi-Impatient Woman and have fairly regular, average-length cycles, you can consider skipping ovulation prediction to follow what I like to call the Lots of Sex Plan (loved by husbands everywhere). Let's say your cycles are normally between 26 and 32 days long. You'll want to have sex every other day between days 7 and 21 of your cycle. That makes it very likely that you will have sex on one of the most fertile days. You don't have to do it every day, as there are two very fertile days in every cycle, but if you leave three days between, you could miss the best opportunity—that's why every other day works best. Every day also works but can get tiring. Contrary to popular belief, male fertility does *not* suffer if you have sex every day (though you might want to hide this bit of information from your husband).

But what if you have more irregular cycles or have regular ones and want to give yourself the best possible chance of getting pregnant? Or what if you just can't fit in that much sex? You'll want to try to predict your most fertile days, which are the two days before ovulation.

There are three primary ways to tell when you ovulate or are about to ovulate: charting, ovulation predictor kits, and fertility monitors. Each has advantages and disadvantages. A lot of books recommend only one of the methods and criticize the others (often unfairly, in my opinion). I think it's better to know about all of the methods and choose the one that will work best for you given your preferences, schedule, financial resources, and cycles. Plus, if you're a Really Impatient Woman, you can use two or even all three of the methods in combination to increase the odds even more.

Charting Your Cycles

Want to learn about your body and find the best days to get pregnant for less than $20? Learn how to chart your cycles using your waking temperature and cervical mucus. Even if you're going to use one of the higher-tech methods, charting can give you useful information about your fertility. You do have to be comfortable touching the stuff that comes out of your vajay-jay, though, and some women think it's messy. (Of course, if you're going to have a baby, you'll be touching stuff a lot messier and stinkier than cervical mucus.) This method also takes some experimenting and learning—though you're learning about your own body, so it's kind of cool.

When I first heard about charting, I thought it was the same as the rhythm method, where couples count days from past cycles to find fertile and infertile days. (Know what you call a man who uses the rhythm method? Daddy.) I'd also heard that taking your temperature to predict ovulation doesn't work because the rise in temperature happens after ovulation and not before, and that the slight dip in temperature before ovulation is too subtle to be useful. But I'd heard wrong on both counts: Charting has nothing to do with the rhythm method, and it uses more than just temperature. I'll give you the basics, and you can get more detail from the excellent book *Taking Charge of Your Fertility* (sometimes abbreviated TCOYF).

The most important aspect of charting for getting pregnant is paying attention to your cervical mucus. Have you ever gone to the bathroom and seen some stretchy clear stuff coming out of you? More than likely, that was cervical mucus flowing out of your vagina, and it's perfectly normal. In fact, it's the best natural sign of fertility. A few days before ovulation, women's bodies make mucus that resembles the clear part of raw eggs in consistency and stretchiness. Egg-white mucus is like a little highway for sperm—they get in it and happily zip along (probably well above the speed limit. Boys!). Sperm die pretty quickly if there's no cervical mucus to help them along—it's as if our bodies tell them not tonight, honey, I'm not fertile yet.

A day or two after your period ends, start checking for

cervical mucus once a day. (Only do this if you are off the pill and preferably have been off it for at least a month, as it can cause mucus to be scant or nonexistent.) Some women check for mucus by looking at the toilet paper after they pee. Others touch the lips of the vagina to feel for mucus. If you want to make sure you're not missing the mucus, you can put a finger into your vagina to check farther up. (Wash your hands first, and don't do it at all if you have long fingernails.) You won't see much those first few days after your period ends. Then you might see white, creamy mucus, and finally, somewhere between 2 and 6 days before you're going to ovulate (often around day 10 if you have an average-length cycle), you'll see clear to whitish watery stuff that will stretch between your fingers and will look like raw egg whites. This is your body's signal that it's time to get it on. You'll see this type of mucus for several days—the average is about five—and then it will disappear, either on the day of ovulation or the day afterward. One study found that sex on days with eggwhite mucus is twice as likely to result in a pregnancy than sex on days with less fertile mucus; another found it was 12 times as likely!

What if you don't see much mucus? Don't panic too soon. Some women only see mucus if they check inside the vagina—and that's okay, because that's where it needs to be. If you've just come off the pill or birth-control shots or just stopped breastfeeding, it will take some time for your mucus to return to normal. Try not to obsess about how much egg-white you get and for how long. You might have only one day, but that's enough to get pregnant. Mucus is not a contest.

Though it can be funny. Patty Debano, one of the authors

of a memoir called *The Conception Chronicles*, remembers reading a book that said, "Be aware of your vagina throughout your cycle." Patty thought this was pretty funny, writing, "Patty could honestly say she had neglected her vagina up until that point, but once she was aware of the daily changes happening in her body, her vagina became a top priority."

The difficulty is that sometimes your vagina is speaking a foreign language and is hard to understand. Most women who chart find that their cycles aren't as perfect as the ones in the TCOYF book. My number of days of eggwhite varied widely, from two to seven, so it wasn't as precise an indicator of impending ovulation as I would have liked. And sometimes it's confusing to interpret the mucus—you have to play the "Is this really eggwhite?" game. If you're tempted to take pictures of your mucus (or take pictures and then post them online), that's a good sign you've gone too far. You might want to stop talking to your vagina for a while or use another method like Ovulation Predictor Kits (OPKs) or a fertility monitor. If you've tried to get pregnant for a few cycles already and rarely see any fertile mucus, consider trying Mucinex or plain cough syrup—both are designed to make mucus more fluid. What works for mucus in the nose and throat may also work for mucus elsewhere. Another alternative is PreSeed—a lubricant that's supposed to mimic eggwhite, and the only lubricant that doesn't kill sperm.

Most women who chart also take their temperature every morning before they get out of bed (basal body temperature or BBT). That's because a woman's temperature rises after she ovulates: After ovulation, the body produces more progesterone, which increases body temperature. Most women

use a digital thermometer, often a special ovulation thermometer that reads to the hundredths of a degree. (You can
buy these online for about $15.) Here's the challenging part:
You'll get the most accurate readings if you take your temperature at the same time every day (including weekends)
and after you've slept (without getting up) for at least three
hours. I've found I can still see a temperature pattern even
when my wake-up times differ by two or three hours, but the
chart is easier to interpret if my wake-up times are the same.

The last day of lower temperatures is usually the day
of ovulation, and the first day of higher temperatures is the
day after. Your temperature will probably stay high until
the first day of your period. That's always been my favorite part about charting—I could predict when my period
would come based on my usual luteal phase and my temperature. When I get a low temperature near the end of
my cycle, my period usually comes that day, so I can pack
supplies, get out the period panties, and not be unpleas-
antly surprised by Aunt Flo (especially useful when teach-
ing classes of 400 students).

You should be able to see ovulation using your temperature, but don't panic if your chart doesn't look as pretty
as the ones in the TCOYF book. The temperature rise after
ovulation can be slow or subtle. Some friends of mine
have never been able to see a temperature rise, yet—given
their several children—are clearly ovulating. Most women,
though, will be able to figure out within a day or two when
and if they ovulated. I pinpointed an ovulation day in about
80 percent of my cycles, but the other 20 percent left me
guessing. Charting has worked very well for both birth con-

trol and fertility for me: I've now charted for seven years, with no unplanned pregnancies and three planned ones.

Because your temperatures show that ovulation has already occurred, they are not useful for timing sex during that cycle. But looking at your temperature pattern over several cycles can give you an idea of when you usually ovulate. It's also the only way to show that you actually did ovulate. OPKs and fertility monitors are good at predicting ovulation by detecting the surge of luteinizing hormone (LH) that occurs a day or two before ovulation. But you won't know how long after the LH surge you ovulate unless you chart your temperature. And on rare occasions, women get an LH surge but don't ovulate.

It's easiest to see the pattern of temperatures if they are on a graph. You can make a graph yourself or get one out of a book. Most have numbers you can circle for the common range of temperatures between 97°F and 100°F. Many women chart online at sites like FertilityFriend.com or tcoyf.com. These sites will also analyze the temperatures and put a little egg on your chart at the most likely day of ovulation. Doing them online allows you to share them with others on message boards. You can also show your pretty-looking charts to your husband, who will feign interest, and your friends, who will either help you obsessively analyze them or will feign interest slightly more convincingly than your husband. I once showed my chart to a neighbor, who was also charting, to get her advice—and then realized that the chart had a little X for every time we had sex. Major overshare. Thankfully, she moved to New Jersey a few months later.

You may or may not want to show your chart to your doctor. Some doctors welcome the opportunity to study your chart with you, but others are skeptical of charting and will even roll their eyes if you talk about it. Some doctors believe that charting is subjective or inaccurate (even though it's not—several journal articles have shown that cervical mucus is a great predictor of fertility). Other doctors think women stress out too much while charting and thus think charting might harm fertility. As you know, studies show that a low to moderate level of stress (and the stress of charting is pretty low) doesn't affect fertility. Many doctors advise against charting because the vast majority of young women get pregnant within a year even without it, but they don't seem to understand that waiting a year—or even three months—is much more stressful than a little charting obsessiveness.

With that said, if you are truly unhappy when you're charting because you're obsessing over it too much, take a cycle or two off and see if you feel better when you're not tracking your ovulation. If you like charting, keep doing it, but just don't tell your doctor about it if he disapproves. Hannah's doctor advised her not to chart, but she continued anyway: "It was because of charting that I realized after two cycles that I ovulated late *and* got my period six days after I ovulated. In other words, it would have been impossible for me to get pregnant. I was able to make an appointment with an RE [reproductive endocrinologist] right away. Had I followed the advice of my OB [obstetrician], I would have waited a full year and would still be TTC instead of holding my baby."

Near the end of your cycle, your temperature might give you an early indication that you're pregnant, rising again about 9 to 12 days after ovulation. This pattern can be subtle, plus not every pregnant woman gets the higher level of temperatures. So to have any certainty you'll still want to take a pregnancy test (see Chapter 8 for the best time to test). Some women continue to chart their temperatures even after they get a positive pregnancy test, because falling temperatures can be an indicator of miscarriage. This can make you crazy really quickly, though, because temperatures are somewhat ambiguous. Sometimes a lower temp means something and sometimes it doesn't. I've seen it go both ways: A lower temp once gave me about eight hours advance notice that I was miscarrying, but I also got a lower temp in my next pregnancy, which produced my full-term daughter. Several lower temps in a row are a more certain indicator that something might be wrong. After you get a positive pregnancy test, you might want to set the thermometer aside to avoid those heart-stopping moments when you are hyperventilating at 5am trying to read your thermometer in the dark.

Ovulation Predictor Kits

Before you started trying to get pregnant, you probably peed on very few things other than a toilet seat (and if you peed on more interesting things, I don't want to know about it). Now that you want to have a baby, you will have the joy of peeing on sticks on a regular basis. Ovulation predictor kits (OPKs) work by detecting luteinizing hormone

(LH), which your body secretes about 32 hours before you ovulate. (It can be anywhere from 12 hours to 48 hours.) You can get OPKs at drugstores, grocery stores, and online. Most kits from stores have five or seven sticks in a box, about a month's supply; they cost between $15 and $30 a box. Online, you can buy the sticks individually for about $2 each. If you have irregular cycles, you'll probably need more than seven sticks per cycle. Several studies and a *Consumer Reports* review found that the most sensitive OPK is the ClearPlan Easy Ovulation Test Pack.

To figure out what day to start testing, begin with the length of your shortest natural cycle (on the pill doesn't count) in the past six months. Then subtract 17 days. (So a woman with a 27-day cycle would start testing on day 10). You'll want to use the OPK between 10am and 8pm, because the LH surge usually shows up in pee during daylight hours. If you can't test at work, testing when you get home (5pm or 6pm) also works. Some women test twice a day so that they don't miss the LH surge, which lasts less than a day.

Reading the tests is a little tricky. For an OPK result to be positive, the test line has to be *darker* than the control line. Just getting a line isn't enough. Many women find that the test line grows steadily darker over a day or two, but the test isn't considered positive until the line is darker than the control. In some ways this is good—a line that's not as dark as the control could tell you you're likely to get a positive soon. If you find the line tests hard to read, buy digital ovulation tests. They are considerably more expensive, but the results are much easier to interpret. (One brand displays a little smiley face for a positive result.) Once you get a positive OPK result, you're done testing for that cycle. (So when do you have sex? See the next chapter.)

Fertility Monitors

If you want a method that takes the guesswork out of finding your fertile time, consider buying a fertility monitor. (The most common is the Clearblue Easy.) You pee on a stick (one especially made for the monitor) every morning and put the stick into a slot in the monitor. It then tells you if your fertility is low, high, or peak. (The last is helpfully indicated with a little egg.) It works by measuring both estrogen and LH. Many women find it easier than OPKs because the monitor tells you whether it needs a stick, reads it, and then displays low, high, or peak on the screen. You don't have to squint at lines, there's no guessing when to test, and it doesn't let you cheap out by trying to use only a few sticks. (I did this when I used OPKs. I thought I knew my cycle well enough to save a few bucks on sticks, but I still missed ovulation more than once.) Some women find it convenient that the monitor uses first morning pee, so they can use it when they're still at home and not yet caught up in the day.

The monitor gives you more information than OPKs because it can identify a longer fertile period (what it calls "high," when it detects more estrogen; this period lasts one to six days and occurs before "peak" fertility). Sometimes the most fertile period has already passed once an OPK turns positive or the egg shows on the monitor. So knowing about those high days is a big plus. Most women don't get a "high" reading until they've already had two or more days of eggwhite, so the monitor gives more precision than charting alone. The user's manual for the monitor also says it will "learn about your cycle" over time, which sounds slightly creepy. As far as I can tell, that just means it asks for fewer sticks as it "learns" the length of your cycle. Some couples wish the monitor computer could perform other functions, too—my friend Michelle's husband thought it should play Marvin Gaye's "Let's Get It On" when it showed "peak" fertility.

The Clearblue Easy monitor costs about $150 to $200, and you also have to buy the special sticks ($35 to $50 for about a three-month supply—most women buy them online). It's much cheaper than most kinds of fertility treatment but much more expensive than charting. One way to save money is to stop using the sticks once you get one "peak" reading. After that, the monitor goes on automatic pilot and will give you another day of peak and one day of high no matter what—even though it asks for them, it doesn't actually read the sticks after giving you the first "egg." (The manual specifically says it will give "peak" the day after the LH surge, and "high" the day after that.)

Using the monitor is a somewhat amusing experience. You put the stick in the machine, wait five interminable minutes, watch it flash a mysterious red light, and then see your fertility level. The waiting can make you a little crazy, as can seeing a result you don't like. Once, when I was impatient to ovulate and the monitor showed low fertility, I flipped it off (and then immediately started laughing at myself). I also learned how to read the sticks myself. The first line is the estrogen reading (which it uses to tell you "high" fertility), and it turns positive when it's *lighter*. The second line is for LH (for "peak"), and it's positive when it's *darker*. The LH line is pretty easy to read, but the estrogen line changes are more subtle and probably best left to the monitor. Still, there were a few times when the monitor read low and I thought it should have said high—and I was right, because peak showed the next day. One of these times led to my third child, which is further proof that being obsessive does have its benefits! (And that cycles that go straight from low to peak can still be fertile.)

A lot of women want to know if it's okay to buy or borrow a used monitor. I think it is even though the company says it's not—but then, they make more money if everyone buys a new one. The pee sticks are capped before they're put into the slot, so there's unlikely to be any contamination (plus it's not like you're going to lick the test slot or something). If you get a used monitor, you should try to reset the memory (search online for how to do this). And don't believe it when they say you have to use sticks from the same pack for each cycle. The Clearblue helpline now says you can use sticks from different packs.

The reviews of the Clearblue monitor on amazon.com, drugstore.com, and other websites will make a believer out of you. Most go like this: "My wife and I tried to get pregnant for a year before we bought this. During the first month, we realized that she was ovulating later than we thought. The second month using this, we got pregnant." Another woman wrote, "Getting my first daughter was supereasy. . . . Now my beautiful princess is 3 and she wants a baby sister, so we took her orders. But we tried for one whole year and nothing happened. I bought some [OPKs], used them occasionally, and they didn't really help. . . . So I got this monitor. It is expensive, with [the] additional cost for test sticks. But it accurately tells me what stage my body is [in] and keeps me testing every day. And I got pregnant during the second [month]." My favorite review was from the man who said the monitor worked "too well." His wife got pregnant on the first cycle. He was "looking forward to at least a month or two of hard work, but instead my part was done before I ever really got started." Poor guy.

I used charting with occasional OPKs to get pregnant the first time and used the monitor for our second and third tries. It was much easier to identify the most fertile days right before ovulation than it was with just charting, and I think it made a difference in getting pregnant fairly quickly in my late 30s. The monitor works well for women of all ages, but it's especially helpful for older women, since we need to make the most of our opportunities. Some of us even get a little attached to our monitors; I saw one post on a message board in which a woman referred to her monitor as "Monnie." When you've nicknamed your fertility monitor, you are truly an Impatient Woman.

Read the Clearblue Easy user's manual for the monitor carefully. The trickiest part is setting the six-hour "testing window" for when you'll pee on your stick in the morning. On the Clearblue Easy, you do this when you press the "m" button at the beginning of your cycle. You should plan carefully when you press that button, because the monitor will set your testing window to be three hours before and three hours after that time. Don't just press it anytime you remember on the first day of your period! (If you do, you can reset it the next morning.) If you usually get up around 7am, pressing it then will give you a window of 4am to 10am. If you sometimes sleep in on the weekends, you might want to press the button later to give you a later window. (Note that you can set the window anytime during the first 5 days of your cycle.) Once the testing window is set for a cycle, you can't change it—which becomes relevant if you travel to another time zone or change your schedule. So try to figure out the earliest and latest time you're likely to test and press the button right in the middle of that window. For example, if you live on the East Coast and are going to be traveling to California, you might want to press the button later than usual. This might involve bringing it to work. I'm hoping future versions of the monitor will find a way around this silliness. (Why doesn't it let you input a time instead of having to press a button at a certain time?) Another way to get around time zone problems is to pee in a cup when you first wake up and then dip the test stick during the next testing window. Just make sure you keep the cup where no one will drink it!

A newcomer to the ovulation predictor business is the OV watch, which detects levels of chloride in your sweat. Chloride levels dip about four days before ovulation and then rise again. Like the fertility monitor, the OV watch can give you more warning of impending ovulation than OPKs. The company says the OV watch increases pregnancy rates 66 percent over OPKs, but I couldn't find any research documenting this. The watch might be worth considering, though, since you don't have to pee on sticks and don't have to designate a testing time as you do with the fertility monitor. You're supposed to wear the watch while you're sleeping, which might be bothersome, but at least you don't have to wear a digital readout of your fertile days on your wrist during the day like a TTC nerd. Another downside is you have to buy a separate supply of sensors, similar to the test sticks for the fertility monitor, and they are more expensive than the fertility monitor sticks. (Sensors are $40 a month—for that, you can get three months of monitor sticks.) On the upside, you only need to wear the watch a few days per cycle, because once it shows the first fertile day, it goes on autopilot and counts down the days to ovulation (it gives four fertile days before O-day). Some women say that the sensors don't work well, though.

Combining the Methods

If you are a Very Impatient Woman, it's possible to use all three methods at once. Before the Merely Impatient But Not Crazy among you laugh, there are some real advantages to this. Fertility monitors are the most foolproof of the three methods, but occasionally—around 3 percent of the time—they will give a too-early false positive for peak fertility. Because the fertility monitor stops measuring anything after you get one peak day, you'll think you ovulated when you didn't and might miss a later ovulation. OPKs also give false positives about 7 percent of the time, and most women stop testing after they get a positive. In both cases, charting will show if you actually ovulated. Fertility monitors can also, though rarely, miss an LH surge and never give you peak fertility. So OPKs can serve as a backup for that scenario. OPKs also have the advantage of use any time of day. You'll want to jump in the sack as soon as you see "peak" fertility on the monitor, so it's inconvenient that you're getting this information first thing in the morning when you're probably blurry-eyed, stinky-breathed, and maybe late for work. OPKs, more commonly used in the afternoon, might warn you with enough time to make dinner plans and, more important, after-dinner plans. You can also use fewer OPK sticks with the fertility monitor because you can wait to test until "high" fertility. But OPKs don't give you the multiple-day opportunities afforded by the monitor, and only charting can tell you if and when you actually ovulated. So using all three methods = not necessarily crazy, and maybe even very smart.

Strength (and Sometimes Stress) in Information

Our husbands, friends, and mothers often see us Impatient Women as obsessive for trying to pinpoint when we ovulate. But having this information can be extremely useful for a number of reasons. Most important, you'll know exactly when you need to have sex to conceive quickly (more on that in the next chapter). And if you know when you ovulated, you will know your exact due date when you get pregnant. Because most women don't know when they ovulate, doctors assume a day 14 ovulation when calculating due dates, but that can be off by days or weeks if you ovulated on a different day of your cycle. Early ultrasounds can peg due dates fairly precisely, but sometimes different ultrasounds give different due dates and doctors will keep moving the date around. This might seem unimportant, as few babies arrive on their exact due dates, but it can be crucial information if your OB wants to induce your labor or schedule a C-section. Even a few days can make a difference between going into labor naturally and being induced for an "overdue" baby who's actually right on time.

Erin relied on the usual day 14 ovulation due date, which for her was March 28. When she said she'd charted and knew she ovulated around day 23 instead, I told her there was no way she was due before the first week of April. By April 1, Erin was upset to be "overdue." Her doctor scheduled an induction, but when she got to the hospital she was already in active labor. Her baby was born on April 7, almost exactly on her real due date by ovulation. I was immature enough to say, "See, I told you so!"

Not all stories have happy endings like Erin's, though. Many women who are induced end up having a C-section, and babies born only a week early are more likely to have trouble breathing. Most "overdue" babies aren't overdue at all, just the product of late ovulations, and that can lead to needless interventions. Doctors these days rarely let you go much beyond 41 weeks (one week beyond the due date), and many start talking about induction at 40 weeks or even earlier. Late in my second pregnancy, my doctor suggested scheduling a C-section in case I went overdue. Happily, I had the baby before that, and without surgery. The next morning, the ringing phone woke up my husband at home. It was the nurse calling to schedule my C-section. "I don't think she needs it," my husband quipped. If my due date had been off by a week or so, it's very possible I would have had an unnecessary C-section.

Tracking your ovulation can also tell you the length of your luteal phase—the days after ovulation but before your next period. The average is 14 days. If your luteal phase is 10, 11, or 12 days, that's on the short side but is usually not a fertility problem. If your luteal phase is 9 days or shorter, it's more likely to be a problem. If you have short luteal phases, try to get pregnant for a few cycles. If you have no luck after four cycles with sex timed around ovulation, consider making a doctor's appointment to talk about taking progesterone. (You have to get this by prescription—the online creams don't work.) Some doctors will also prescribe Clomid, an ovulation drug, to lengthen a short luteal phase (see Chapter 10).

A surprising cause of short luteal phases for some women is exercise, particularly running. If you're a runner, you might want to taper down your miles before trying to get pregnant. Short luteal phases are also more common as you get older, and they are virtually guaranteed when your fertility is resetting itself—after having a baby, breastfeeding, or the first cycle or two after coming off the pill.

Medical researchers disagree about short luteal phases: Some say they aren't a problem for fertility and others say they are but that they're caused by a weak egg, not by low progesterone alone. (That's why Clomid, which produces a "stronger" ovulation, is often prescribed.) When I first started charting, I noticed right away that I had a short luteal phase, usually only 11 days and sometimes only 10. I still don't know why. Fortunately, I got pregnant with my first daughter unassisted. The second time around, I was freaked out because my luteal phase was even shorter—only 9 days and sometimes just 8. I then had an early miscarriage and wondered if the short luteal phase had caused it. So when I got pregnant again, I started taking progesterone a few days after the positive test. I might not have needed it— my blood progesterone levels tested just fine, and most of the time, if a healthy embryo implants, it sends a signal to keep the cycle going. (The medical journals use the chivalrous term *corpus luteum rescue*.) But the embryo still needs enough time to implant, and according to the best research study, most embryos implant on days 8, 9, or 10 after ovulation. So an 8-day luteal phase could definitely hamper fertility, and a 9-day might. But definitely not always—just ask my second child. (I did. She said, "Ga." I assume that's baby for "I kicked that short luteal phase right in the butt.")

It is sometimes difficult to strike a balance between knowing too little and knowing too much about your fertility. Charting, OPKs, and fertility monitors can fuel obsessiveness about getting pregnant, which can become all-consuming. "I've been taking my temperature every morning for over a year," says Britney, 30. "I wake up all through the night anticipating my 5:15am alarm that signals permission to take another temperature reading. One high temp has me eagerly anticipating the passing of the next 24 hours, when I can hopefully chart another one, potentially signaling pregnancy. My husband now requests a temperature report each morning; it's become quite an obsession for both of us." OPKs, and especially the fertility monitor, can also cause a lot of anxiety. It's easy to worry if you're not getting high fertility and then to worry again if you're not getting peak fertility. Once you get the little egg, you worry that you might not have had sex early enough. There's also an illogical but overwhelming feeling of suspense after you put your stick into the machine and it blinks for five minutes before displaying the reading. I can remember my heart beating really fast when I was waiting for the results, as if I were getting my SAT scores back. There was no rational reason to be nervous about it, but I was anyway. If you feel yourself getting nervous at these times, turn to Chapter 7 for ways to calm down—especially the sections on relaxation techniques and ruminating.

Ovulation Prediction While Breastfeeding

Ovulation prediction can be more difficult if you are breastfeeding or recently weaned a baby. If you're breastfeeding a baby who's less than 6 months old and not supplementing with formula, you probably haven't ovulated yet and thus are very unlikely to get pregnant. You'll start ovulating and then get a period once your baby starts solid food or formula and is nursing less. For some women, this happens within a few months of their baby eating other food; for others, their periods might not return until the baby is fully weaned. My periods came back when my daughter was 9 months old and eating lots of baby food, even though she was still nursing four times a day. These cycles were wacky, though, with almost undetectable temperature rises and really short luteal phases. My cycles got back to normal about three months after I stopped breastfeeding, which is about the average. Mother Nature apparently wants kids to be spaced at least two years apart, and indeed that's what happens in cultures where women breastfeed their children and don't use any other birth control.

So if you're trying to get pregnant when you're breast-feeding, expect some challenges. After your period returns, OPKs and fertility monitors should be able to detect your ovulation, but charting might reveal scant fertile mucus and very short luteal phases. It's certainly possible to get preg-nant while breastfeeding, but if you're serious about getting pregnant quickly, you'll want to wait until you've weaned your baby and probably a few cycles afterward. I know this can be tough—both you and your baby probably love nurs-ing. The day I wrote this, I breastfed my 12-month-old for the last time, and even thinking about that makes me cry (although she has six teeth now—that also made me cry while breastfeeding, but for different reasons).

Or maybe you're looking forward to weaning, and wanting to get pregnant again is another good reason to stop. You probably already know all of the reasons to keep breastfeeding until at least a year, but if you've made it to six months, that's really great, too. Especially if you're back to working full-time, pumping can be a real pain (literally and figuratively), so wanting to wean is understandable.

Now, the chapter you've been waiting for. When, and how, should you have sex while trying to conceive?

CHAPTER 4

Horizontal Mambo: The Best Time to Dance the Baby Dance

Now that you know how to predict when you're going to pop out an egg, how do you get the sperm there to meet it? Well, the *how* part you already know—you get laid, make love, shag, roll in the hay, get it on, or whatever creative name you find by Googling "synonyms for sex." (Try it—you'll see some you've never heard and others you wish you never had.) When trying to conceive, some women call sex baby dancing, or BDing for short. For getting pregnant, the key is *when* you dance.

When you were younger, or just started having sex with your man, or didn't already have a child (or a job), or simply had more time, the question of when to have sex wasn't really an issue, because you did it all the time—once a day, sometimes twice on the weekends. If you still have sex this often, you can skip this chapter.

(Pause.)

Now that the 99.5 percent of you who are from planet Earth are still with me, let's talk about the best time to have sex if you want to get pregnant. Timing sex is more important than most people realize. At most, only six days of your monthly cycle are at all fertile, and only two of them are the most fertile. So if you're having sex once a week without any consideration of when you ovulate, you'll probably miss these days completely. If you're having sex twice a week, you're still likely to miss the best two days. And if you're having sex less than once a week: First, welcome to the silent sisterhood, and second, don't worry—you can get pregnant from having sex just once a month, as long as it's on the right day (though two days is better, and trying to get pregnant is a great excuse to revive your sex life). If you're even a little impatient to get pregnant quickly, timing is everything. Many couples who try for months without success are just timing things wrong.

Most books, Internet sites, and OPK or fertility monitor instruction sheets say that the day you ovulate is the most fertile. But the latest research, based on four different studies, shows that the most fertile days are one and two days before ovulation. For women in their late 20s and early 30s, the chance of getting pregnant on the day of ovulation is less than 1 in 10, but two days before ovulation it's 1 in 3— *three times* higher! You can up those chances even more if you have sex more than once during your fertile time.

So why is the day of ovulation *not* the most fertile? It's probably because of the short life of the egg, only 6 to 12 hours. Especially if you're having sex in the evening—and that's the norm for most couples—you might miss the egg entirely, or at least miss the time when it's most likely to lead to a healthy pregnancy. The best-known study of natural fertility originally showed high fertility for the day of ovulation (which is probably how this rumor got started).

But when the researchers looked at which pregnancies survived past 6 weeks, they found that a large percentage of conceptions from sex on the day of ovulation led to early miscarriages. So having sex on the days before ovulation and not just on the day of ovulation is an effective way to lower your risk of an early miscarriage. So don't make the mistake of waiting too long to baby dance.

When to Have Sex to Boost Your Chances of Getting Pregnant

The difficulty is you won't know which days are one and two days before ovulation until after you've ovulated. Making your best guess for these days depends on which method of ovulation prediction you're using and how much time and enthusiasm you have for sex. The first option is the husband-approved Lots of Sex Plan I mentioned in the previous chapter, having sex every other day between day 7 and day 20 of your cycle. (This only works if you have regular cycles between 26 and 32 days long.) You might have heard it's better to have sex spaced several days apart so that the man's sperm count doesn't go down. Research doesn't bear this out—even men with a low sperm count are just as fertile with daily sex. Sex every other day during the fertile period will work almost as well in terms of getting pregnant, but if you'd rather indulge every night, go for it.

If you want to be more precise and aim for the most fertile days, your chosen method of ovulation prediction will help you. If you're charting your cycles, have sex the first day you see eggwhite mucus and then every day or every other day until your temperature rises. If you want to narrow things down further and you've charted for a few cycles already, count the number of days of eggwhite you usually have so that you can try to peg the magic one or two days before ovulation. A FertilityFriend.com study of 119,398 charts showed that 94 percent of pregnancies occurred from sex on the three days around ovulation (the two days before and the day of).

If you're using OPKs, hop in the sack on the first day you get a positive. Then have sex again the next day, just to cover the bases. The downside of OPKs is you get only a few hours of warning for your highest fertility, which can make it harder to plan ahead. Some women (including me) don't get a positive until the day of ovulation, which is already past the most fertile time. Some women notice over several cycles that they get a faint line before they get a darker, truly positive line, and that gives them a warning of about a day.

With the Clearblue Easy fertility monitor, the "high" days give you even more warning time. But even though the digital readout seems so trustworthy, you'll have to adjust your thinking to use it most effectively. The monitor's symbols and user manual assume that the day of ovulation is the most fertile even though it's not. Ovulation usually occurs between 8 and 24 hours after the "peak" egg shows up on the monitor. So the true two days of peak fertility are the last day of "high" and the first day of "peak." If you wait for "peak" fertility, especially if you're baby dancing at night, you may have already missed the most fertile time. You've almost certainly missed it if you wait until the second "peak" day (which really shouldn't be labeled that way).

Women in one study used the Clearblue monitor and had an ultrasound every morning to pinpoint the day of ovulation. About 15 percent of the time, ovulation occurred before the morning ultrasound on the first peak day. And 76 percent of the time it had occurred by the morning of the second peak day. With the day of ovulation less fertile, 91 percent of women have exited their most fertile time by the second peak day, and 15 percent are already out of it by the first peak day. So if you're charting as well as using the monitor, you're most likely to get the first peak reading on your last day of low temperature (not the second-to-last day, as you might expect). Once you've used the monitor for a cycle or two, you might know how many days of "high" you usually get. *Aim to have sex on the last day of "high" and the first day of "peak."* For most women, the second "peak" day and the "high" afterward are already past the most fertile time. If the second peak day is your only choice, it's still worth trying, but your chances will be less. For both peak days, sex in the morning is more likely to catch the egg.

How to Have Sex to Boost your Chances of Getting Pregnant

Reproductive sex can be really fun—there's no worrying about the condom breaking, no pills to take, and a beautiful sense of purpose to it all. The challenge is that having sex spontaneously and randomly twice a week might not get you pregnant as quickly as sex timed around ovulation, and having sex only once a week might mean waiting two to three times as long to get pregnant. So you have to find some way to make sex fun and relatively spontaneous even though it's the fertility monitor—and not your libido—that's telling you to head for the bedroom.

So even when the fertility monitor pops up the egg and your brain is screaming, "It has to be tonight! This is it!" it's better to put on the lingerie and drop subtle hints. Resist the urge to rotate your hips and suggestively wave your OPK stick. Anything you just peed on is not romantic.

Unfortunately, husbands—the usual sex instigators—are blissfully ignorant about the most fertile times to have sex. More than likely, your husband has memorized the NBA playoff schedule but has no clue where you are in your monthly cycle—yes, even if you've been talking about it constantly. (This is called selective deafness. It's also the reason he didn't hear you when you asked him to take out the trash.) There's a chance you might be able to get him interested in the statistics here—compare them to batting averages or something (that is, assuming you weren't selectively deaf when he spent an hour explaining them to you). Guys love sports stats, and sex stats aren't all that far off. Of course, he might end up bragging about it to his buddies: "Sex in my house is up 40 percent from two months ago! Whoo!"

One Impatient Woman's husband asked her to promise six months of "practicing trying to conceive" before they actually started trying. "That's right," she says, "six months of pretending to get pregnant so that he could reap the benefits of extra sex." Stacy says, "My husband interpreted every single question I asked him as a euphemism for sex! I heard, 'Is that a euphemism?' countless times during the week."

After you've been trying for a few months, sex on demand gets difficult. It's like being in a weekly porn movie where you have to perform as soon as the director (in this case, the fertility monitor) says, "Action!" You're tired of it, and he feels like a sperm donor. Elizabeth, 41, says, "God, sex just sucked while trying to get pregnant—how ironic." Another woman, who got pregnant with twins after years of infertility, remarked to a friend with relief, "And now we never have to have sex again."

It's tough to remember to just have fun. Try not to put him on too precise a schedule. Yes, he needs to know how important timing is, but the more times you can entice him without explicitly announcing your ovulation, the better. For the average guy, all it takes is leading him to the bedroom or looking at him pointedly when you take off your shirt. *The Conception Chronicles* author Patty Debano says that when she first started using OPKs, she laughed and said to her husband, "If the stick is blue, you know what to do." After six months of this, though, she would wave the stick in her husband's face and yell, "Come on!" as she ran to the bedroom. Finally, she bought lingerie that "could double as a rock-climbing harness."

Fortunately, even sex on demand can be fun once you've started. Just take it slow at first and try to concentrate on the positive feelings in the present moment. Wanting to have a baby might be the reason you start, but it shouldn't be what you're thinking about during. Even if you weren't in the mood before you started, you can take pleasure in it.

Don't use lubricants like K-Y jelly, Astroglide, scented oils, spit, or even water. All of them can kill sperm. If you can go natural, that's best—foreplay helps. (Yes! An excuse for foreplay!) If you need some extra help, you can try a lubricant called PreSeed that more closely resembles natural lubrication and doesn't kill sperm. Some women use PreSeed to enhance their fertility if they think they don't have enough cervical mucus. Others try actual egg whites from eggs. (This runs the risk of salmonella from the raw eggs, though. If you try it, don't forget to warm up the eggs first! Cold things in hoochie = no fun.) As with most supplements and unusual techniques, I think it's best to try the natural way for a few months first.

What do you do with the extra Astroglide? When my dad and I put together a play structure for my daughter, the poles kept sticking in the openings in the tent fabric. I ran up the stairs, grabbed the Astroglide, and boop! in went those poles. (When my mother asked, I told her it was Vaseline.)

Once you've ditched the lubricant, it's time to figure out the best sexual position. I tried to find actual research on sexual positions and pregnancy rates, but there was nothing. Clearly, somebody needs to write a research grant to study this. I've already got the title: "Doin' It Doggy Style or Ridin' It Cowgirl: Which Is More Likely to Put a Bun in the Oven?" Most books say that the missionary position (man on top) is best because the vagina slants toward the cervix in that position, so gravity helps the little swimmers get where they need to go. Woman on top (cowgirl) would thus be less desirable. Of course, unless you're hopping off the horse the second he's done, the little swimmers are presumably on their way anyway. (We really do need a study on this—how hard would it be? Sorry, bad pun.) One Impatient Woman I know tried for six months using the missionary position before switching to doggy style on a whim—and that's when she got pregnant. (She might have had a tipped uterus . . . or it might have been coincidence.) So if one way isn't working, mix it up a little. By then you might welcome the change anyway!

Some books say that you're more likely to get pregnant if the woman has an orgasm, on the theory that this hoovers up the little swimmers. There's no research on that either. Yet another grant proposal I'd like to read: "Does the Oven Have to Climax to Get a Bun in It? A Randomized Controlled Trial."

Should you sit with your legs elevated, with a pillow under your butt (the "bug" position) after sex? No studies on that one either. Some studies show that you're more likely to get pregnant if you stay lying down after sex for at least 15 minutes—that was among women who had intrauterine insemination instead of the fun way, but it still makes sense to not jump up right away. But remember that you don't need to do this in any weird position. Bicycling your legs in the air until the blood rushes to your head isn't necessary, although it is funny.

There actually is one study that shows why position, pillows, and all that doesn't make much difference. The researchers put "technetium-labeled albumin macrospheres of sperm size" (ohhkay) in the back of women's vaginas during their fertile times. Some of the particles found their way to the fallopian tubes—where fertilization usually takes place—within *one* minute. One! I always thought the sperm were chillin' in there for a while, reading little magazines and watching ESPN on tiny TVs. And maybe they do several days before ovulation, but apparently some of them can sprint pretty fast when they have to. Sounds *a lot* like men in general.

You can test this men-are-like-sperm theory by seeing how fast he will race to the bedroom when you suggest you might have a present for him in there—you. Anything, even cheese like this, is a better aphrodisiac than waving an OPK stick and yelling, "Right now! It has to be right now!" It might be sex on demand, but that doesn't mean it can't be fun.

CHAPTER 5

Choosing the Sex
of Your Baby

Would you like to have a girl or a boy? As much as we say we just want a healthy baby (and we do!), most of us can't help wishing for a particular gender. The reasons are as varied as our families. Many women want at least one girl—a companion for girl stuff and someone to wear the adorable girl outfits. Girls are also rumored to be easier—at least until they are teenagers, when boys presumably inspire less parental worry. A lot of men, secretly or not so secretly, really want a boy, especially for a first-born child. Of course, there are also plenty of women who want boys and men who want Daddy's girls. Couples who already have a child or children of one gender often want one of the other gender to "balance" the family. These fervent wishes are very common, despite our guilt about them and the social unacceptability of giving them voice. "Sex preference is more the rule than the exception, no matter what parents say," maintains family therapist Joshua Coleman.

So what can you do if you really want a girl, or really want a boy? Only two techniques have proven success rates over 80 percent: preimplantation genetic diagnosis (PGD; it's used with IVF) and MicroSort.

No, I'm not suggesting Bill Gates choose the sex of your baby. (*That's* an Excel chart I want to see.) MicroSort is a sperm-sorting procedure used by the Genetics and IVF Institute, a Virginia fertility clinic. To use MicroSort, you have to become part of their clinical trial and have an IUI (intrauterine insemination) or use IVF.

The sorting is done using a flow cytometer (which writer Lisa Belkin describes as "a beige box of a machine about the size of an L-shaped office desk that spends all day, every day, sorting sperm"). The woman then receives the sperm using a medicalized version of a turkey baster; apparently, women get to watch via ultrasound as the cloud of sperm races upward. Ninety-three percent of couples who want a girl get one, and 82 percent who want a boy are successful. The researchers have published their results in many medical journal articles. "It's in a different category from everything else," Dr. Alan Copperman, the director of reproductive endocrinology at the Mount Sinai Medical Center, told *The New York Times Magazine* in 1999. "It is not a scam." The MicroSort webpage features a happy family of four, with mom holding the boy and dad the girl.

To use MicroSort, couples must be married, the woman must be age 39 or younger, and the couple should either be a carrier of a sex-linked genetic disease (such as hemophilia) or already have at least one child and want to have a child of the other gender. During the 2000s, most MicroSort patients used the procedure for family balancing, but in 2010 the clinic closed that portion of the clinical trial. As of this writing, MicroSort is only available to couples with risks for genetic diseases (visit www.microsort.net to see the current status, as they may go back to family balancing—there's certainly demand for it). IUIs must be done at one of two sites: Fairfax, Virginia (in the DC suburbs), or Laguna Hills, California (in Orange County, south of Los Angeles). If you're already shelling out the big bucks for IVF, the institute will sort the sperm, freeze it, and ship it on to your location. MicroSort is not cheap. Not including travel to Virginia or Orange County (a "conception tour," as one couple called it), each sort costs $2,995, which insurance does not cover, plus a patient consultation fee of $300, plus the cost of the IUI (often around $400 per attempt). And only 17 percent of women get pregnant per IUI.

The only way to virtually guarantee the sex of a baby is to undergo IVF and use PGD, a procedure that extracts a cell or two from an embryo while it's still floating in a petri dish. The cell's chromosomes are then analyzed, and only the embryos of the desired sex are implanted. Given the ethical issues involved, only some doctors will use this technique for family balancing, though almost all are willing to use it for carriers of sex-linked genetic diseases.

Two other assisted reproduction methods also tilt the sex ratio, but not by much. An IUI with (unsorted) fresh sperm results in a boy baby 56 percent of the time. Taking Clomid results in girl babies 54 percent of the time. The two effects cancel each other out when IUI and Clomid are used together, as they often are in fertility treatment.

Sperm Sorting in the Bedroom: What the Data Say

So what if you really want a boy, or a girl, but don't have the time, money, or eligibility for these medical interventions? What can you try at home to tilt the odds toward the gender of your choice? I was, and still am, very interested in the answer to this question. My husband and I wanted at least two children, and it was my greatest fear that we would have two boys who would inherit my high energy level and pummel each other all day. I also really wanted at least one girl. So when we found out our first child was a girl, I was thrilled. I yelled, "Yes!" and pumped the air as if I'd just caught a touchdown pass. My husband was happy, too, but then he looked worried and said, "Uh-oh. What if she's hot?"

When we found out our second child was also a girl, I was happy, though surprised. I'd avoided pink in everything from car seats to sippy cups in anticipation of the statistically expected boy. I was a little disappointed not to have one of each, and my husband complains about being outnumbered, but I liked the idea of two sisters, having two presumably easier-to-manage children, and reusing all of those cute baby girl clothes. When we were trying for our third (and presumably last) child, I wanted a boy because we could have the experience of both genders without the possibility of my feared two-boys-endlessly-smacking-each-other scenario. It would be the perfect way to have lots of pink cake and eat some blue cake, too (as scared as I still am of seeing my personality combined with higher levels of testosterone). So I've been in the position of both really wanting a girl and really wanting a boy. (So was our third child a boy or a girl? I'll tell you at the end of the chapter.)

The most popular at-home technique for sex selection is promoted by Dr. Landrum Shettles, who wrote *How to Choose the Sex of Your Baby* in 1970. The book was updated in 1996 and 2006, with coauthor David Rorvik, and its cover says it's sold a whopping 1.5 million copies. Because the boy (Y) sperm are lighter, Dr. Shettles theorized, they swim faster and get to the egg first. Thus, having sex close to ovulation should produce more boys. The girl (X) sperm are slower, but live longer, so having sex further from ovulation should produce more girls. Dr. Shettles claimed an 80 percent success rate for his technique based on letters from his readers, and numerous websites and books recommend the technique.

Dr. Shettles' eminently logical theory has just one thing wrong with it: It doesn't work. Eight scientific studies published in medical journals examined sex timing and the baby's gender, and most find the *opposite* of Shettles' theory, with more girls conceived from sex on the day of ovulation and more boys conceived from sex many days before. Why do the letters from Dr. Shettles' readers suggest otherwise? Probably because those who were successful were much more likely to write in, which gives a distorted picture of the results. This may also be why Dr. Shettles never published his data in a medical journal, since reputable journals require studies to be scientific and have unbiased data.

In my day job as a psychology researcher, I often do studies called meta-analyses that combine data over many studies—an effective technique for discovering an overall pattern. So I did that here. Across eight studies with data from 1,672 births, 55 percent of babies from the day of ovulation were girls, compared to 45 percent from 2 or more days before ovulation, with only a 4 in 10,000 probability that the difference was due to chance. On the day before ovulation, there was a roughly even split. At the very least, these data suggest that Shettles' theory is ineffective. (If you're wondering what Dr. Shettles and his coauthor have to say about these studies, see Appendix G.)

An Australian study found that 73 couples who used the Shettles method—following the recommendations for timing, abstinence, and douching according to whether they wanted a son or a daughter—usually got a baby the *opposite* gender from what they wanted. Among those who wanted a son and had sex close to ovulation, 63 percent gave birth to daughters, and of those who wanted a daughter and had sex far from ovulation, 52 percent had sons. A 1995 study of 127 pregnancies found a similar pattern, with 53 percent of ovulation-day babies girls, compared to only 43 percent girls from sex two or more days before ovulation, though this difference was not statistically significant. This study attributed the conception to the sex closest to ovulation (which might not have been true—who knows how the sperm fight it out in there?). That may have muddled the results and pushed them closer to the 50/50 split expected by chance. The results are probably the most reliable for the days furthest away from ovulation, and those days produced 57 percent boys.

One study conducted in New Zealand was especially strong in its research design. It asked couples to have sex on *only* one day during their fertile time, which gives much-needed precision to the results. Ovulation was pinpointed using three different methods: LH from urine samples, the women's reports of cervical mucus, and temperature shift. Couples in the first half of the study used the Shettles timing, and those in the second half did the opposite; that helps rule out the possibility that something about the couples and why they wanted a boy rather than a girl caused the results.

Across 55 births, 90 percent of ovulation-day babies were girls, and only 21 percent of the babies from sex two or more days before ovulation were girls (and thus 79 percent were boys). I reanalyzed the data myself and found that there's less than a 2 in 10,000 probability the difference occurred by chance. These were the results with ovulation measured by LH; using the peak day of mucus or the last day of high temperature yielded the same basic pattern but not as striking.

So the study with the best design found the biggest difference. In research this usually means that there actually *is* a difference, especially since almost all of the studies, even those with inferior research designs, found the same basic pattern. So the timing of sex relative to ovulation does make a difference in influencing the gender of your baby, but the formula is further away for a boy and closer for a girl.

How can this be, when the boy sperm swim faster and the girl sperm live longer? It might have more to do with the survival of the embryo than the sperm. More male than female embryos are conceived, but male embryos are more likely to miscarry, which evens out the sex ratio by birth. That might be why day-of-ovulation babies are so much more likely to be girls: the North Carolina study found that many of these embryos were lost. Those that survive are likely to be the hardier female embryos. Some other factor must favor boy sperm earlier in the cycle. In the end, the *why* doesn't matter much—it's the results, which clearly show more boys from earlier sex and more girls from later.

0+12

Several books and websites tell the (possibly apocryphal) story of Kynzi from Queensland, Australia. Married in 1975, Kynzi and her husband were pleased to welcome two boys to their family in the years after their wedding. They wanted more children and hoped to have a girl. A neighbor told her about the Shettles method, which Kynzi put into practice, having sex three days before ovulation and not after. But she had another boy. She used the technique two more times to try to have a girl, adding douching, diet, and other recommendations, and she had two more boys. Then they tried the Chinese birth chart and had another boy. With six boys, Kynzi and her husband decided to give up, and she made an appointment to have her tubes tied. While waiting for the doctor, she chatted with the nurse about her unusual family of six boys. The nurse searched for some studies on sex selection and found the New Zealand study, which, to Kynzi's shock, showed that timing sex several days away from ovulation was more likely to result in boys—exactly what had happened to her.

Kynzi decided not to have her tubes tied just yet and went home to consider trying one last time to have a girl. Coincidentally, she ovulated that day and laid in bed wondering what to do. In the end, she and her husband decided to go for it. They didn't get much afterglow. Right as they finished, their 5-year-old ran into their room sick to his stomach. (This is my favorite part of the story—there's nothing more romantic than a barfing kindergartener. Isn't it amazing that people who already have kids ever manage to reproduce again?) Despite the barf-fest, Kynzi and her husband got their happy ending in another way: a girl. After her daughter arrived, Kynzi found herself "checking" the baby's diaper in disbelief: Was she still a girl? And when she sent out her Christmas card with the baby dressed in pink lace, her friends asked her to send a picture of the baby with full frontal nudity—since they knew it was Kynzi's last child, they figured that she might even dress a boy that way!

Kynzi's story and the New Zealand data led to some discussion of a girl-achieving method called 0+12, which suggests postponing sex until 12 hours after you ovulate. Does it work? Sort of. The research does suggest that sex the day of ovulation is more likely to result in a girl. But waiting until 12 hours after ovulation isn't a good idea because sex after ovulation is less likely to lead to pregnancy than one or two days before and more likely to lead to early miscarriage. And most studies find *no* pregnancies from sex the day after ovulation. So what can you do?

Sex Timing for Having a Girl Versus a Boy

If you want a girl, time sex as close to ovulation as possible, between 12 hours before and 6 hours after ovulation. If you're using a fertility monitor, that would mean sex on the second day of "peak" fertility (so the second day of getting the "egg")—preferably in the morning to maximize the chance of getting pregnant at all. If you think you usually ovulate within 12 to 18 hours of getting the "egg," try the first day of peak, probably at night. For an OPK the advice is similar—sex the day *after* you get a positive. If you're charting, aim for the day you are guessing will be the last day of low temperature (which might be hard to guess).

If you want a boy, aim to have sex two or three days before ovulation. You'll up your chances of a boy, though lowering your odds of conceiving at all, the more days away from ovulation you get. A compromise is to aim for two days before, which is still very fertile. Pinpointing these days can be tricky. If you're using a fertility monitor, have sex on the "high" fertility days and then stop once you get the egg for "peak." If you're using an OPK, buy an old-fashioned one with lines and not a digital one, and have sex when the line is heading toward being as dark as the control line but hasn't made it yet. Once you get a positive, no more sex. If you're charting, use your past cycles to try to predict what will be two or three days before ovulation. If you usually get four to five days of eggwhite, your best bet for a boy will be the first day or two of eggwhite mucus.

Try any of these only with the realization that you could easily get a child of either gender. Remember that several studies found only a few percentage points difference by timing sex close to or further from ovulation. The New Zealand study did find a bigger difference, with the day of ovulation leading to many more girl babies, but it was a small study. The difference from a 50/50 split was probably not due to chance, but it's still very possible the difference is smaller than what they found or that the couples differed in some way from most couples trying to get pregnant. In addition, ovulation prediction is an inexact science. You don't know for sure which day is, for example, three days before ovulation until it's past. So in real life using sex timing to conceive a child of one gender or the other may be even less effective that these statistics suggest. My guess, based on the data, is that you can probably shift the odds, at most, to about 60 percent. Want to increase your chances even more? Maybe you can eat your way to a boy or a girl.

Preconception Diet and the Sex of Your Baby

Apparently, the key is to eat lots of food if you want to have a boy and less if you want a girl. A 2008 study of 740 normal-weight white British women found that 56 percent of those who were in the top third of calorie consumption (about 2,250 calories a day) had boys, compared to 45 percent in the lowest third (1,750). Women who conceived boys ate more protein, carbohydrates, folate, zinc, iron, sodium, calcium, and potassium. Of 133 specific foods, the largest difference was for breakfast cereal. Among women who regularly ate cereal, 59 percent had boys, compared to 43 percent of those who didn't. The women also reported what they ate in early pregnancy, but that didn't differ, which makes it less likely the preconception diet results were due to something about the women than something about the diet. The authors theorized that humans evolved to have more sons when times were good and food was plentiful.

The weakness of this study is that women who were already three months pregnant were asked to recall what they ate before they got pregnant. I can barely remember what I ate for lunch yesterday, much less three months ago. Yet most people have fairly reliable eating patterns, especially for breakfast, and that's where they found the biggest effect. The other possibility is the difference in diet is just a reflection of differences among the women that might also lead to having more boys versus girls. The women weren't told what to eat, so it's possible that other factors (social class, education, exercise, or something unknown) caused both eating more and being more likely to have a boy. Exercise is a particularly interesting possibility, as the women who had boys ate more calories but were the same weight as those who had girls—and that only seems possible if they exercised more.

A 1980 study also found effects for diet. The researchers spun a hard-to-follow theory about "overcharging the body with potassium ions" to have a boy and undercharging to have a girl. Couples followed a very specific diet one to two months before trying to conceive. The diet was required for the women and suggested for the men "for psychological reasons"—probably because little baby-making and much resentment might occur if the men ate whatever they wanted while the women ate this weird diet. The daily "girl diet" included 1,528 milligrams of calcium, 254 milligrams of magnesium, 675 milligrams of sodium, and 2,947 milligrams of potassium, plus a supplement of 500 milligrams of calcium with vitamin D. The "boy diet" required 297 milligrams of calcium, 135 milligrams of magnesium, 5,000 milligrams of sodium, and 3,873.5 milligrams of potassium, supplemented with 600 milligrams of potassium chloride. The study reported that 80 percent of 260 couples had a baby of the sex they wanted.

These are pretty awesome results, approaching those of MicroSort. Eating differently for a few months doesn't sound too bad. But the dietary requirements are so exact that I'm not sure how anyone could pull them off. The researchers even scolded that the success rate depended on how well the women adhered to the diet, to which I say, "You try it." If you decide to give the diet a shot, you'll probably have to take supplements and find foods that fit the requirements. Potassium-rich foods include bananas, spinach, squash, potatoes, and oranges; calcium-rich foods include milk, cheese, yogurt, and leafy green vegetables.

If you want a girl, it's relatively easy to supplement with an extra calcium tablet a day. But if you want a boy, potassium supplementation is more difficult. Slow-K, the product used in the study, is by prescription only. The alternative is lower-dose supplements of potassium gluconate; I found some at a regular drugstore. I'd also be wary of being on the boy diet for any length of time. Women, especially those trying to get pregnant, need a lot more than 297 milligrams of calcium a day, and 5,000 milligrams of sodium sounds like a festival of potato chips and canned soup, not exactly the picture of health. A diet with that much salt could lead to water retention and more serious complications if you already have high blood pressure. The girl diet seems a little healthier, but get ready to *really* like milk and yogurt.

And keep in mind that the 2008 study instead concluded that the more calories overall, including from calcium, led to boy babies. I'm also skeptical of the 1980 study because so few details are provided in the article: The results section is only two paragraphs long, with no tables or graphs, and the authors don't describe just how the women managed to follow such a complicated diet. But if you really want a girl, or really want a boy, it might be worth trying for a few months. Or you can go with the results of the 2008 study and eat a lot of calories (especially breakfast cereal) if you want a boy and eat fewer calories if you want a girl.

There's one last item worth mentioning for influencing the sex of your child: DHEA, the supplement I mentioned in Chapter 1. At one fertility clinic, 61 percent of women who took DHEA had boy babies, which rose to 69 percent boys among those conceiving naturally. This study was very small, only 31 births, but the results are strong enough to merit consideration of DHEA if you'd like to have a boy (with all of the caveats I mentioned in Chapter 1).

What about combining the sex timing and diet methods? Would that up the chances of getting the girl, or the boy, you want? It might. So have fun trying!

So how did our quest for a boy go? At 39, almost 40, I was afraid I wouldn't get pregnant at all, so we didn't try to sway gender based on timing. I did make some changes to

my diet, scaling back on calcium and taking potassium supplements. I ate my cereal every morning (though I'd done
that with the girls, too). When we got the genetic testing
results back, we were mostly relieved that everything was
normal. Of course, we were also excited to find out the sex:
The baby was a . . . girl.

Internet Methods

You might be tempted to try other gender-swaying methods you've found on the Internet. There's the Chinese Gender Chart, purportedly "found in an ancient royal tomb
near Beijing" (What is that I smell?) and "said to be over 90
percent accurate in predicting your baby's gender." (Beep!
Beep! Beep! There goes my b.s. detector—"said to be" by
whom? Passive voice: the refuge of people who make things
up.) The website The Bump has a particularly cute chart—
enter your age at conception and the month, and it scrolls
down the chart, where a cute little cartoon baby wrapped
in either pink or blue says, "Hi, Mom!" It's so adorable it's a
shame that it's complete hooey.

The site invites readers to comment on whether it
"worked for you," featuring an even split between those
who said it worked and those who didn't. (Not a scientific
sample, but I doubt a researcher will ever do a study to dis-
prove it.) Many women took the chart seriously and planned
their pregnancy attempts around it. "I had my hopes up and
planned around this [to get a girl] and boy number three
is on his way!" said one. "We'll go for a boy when I am 30

because the summer is all blue," noted another. My advice: Don't structure your life around something that somebody made up. Another commenter said, "Yes, it worked for me and it's weird, because I went to one or another website and it said I was having a boy." Because, apparently, several people have made up different versions of this chart that contradict one another. Others pointed out that "you need to find out your Chinese age [based on your own conception, not your birthdate] and the lunar month for the chart to be accurate." So you have to do some weird calculations to make sure you are looking at the right column in something that someone made up.

At least the Chinese Gender Chart is free (or shown after you type in your email address). Several other websites use convincingly scientific language to rake in cash for their gender selection methods. GenSelect ($199 for one month and a whopping $439 for three months) features blue and pink boxes with BOY! and GIRL! written on them, which include nutritional supplement pills, OPKs (presumably to use the disproven Shettles method?), and douching materials (doctors recommend you don't douche, ever, especially when you're trying to get pregnant). The website says the technique "has proven 96 percent effective in controlled studies" and was published in the *Journal of General Medicine*—a journal that is not listed in the comprehensive journal database Medline. Neither is the doctor associated with the site. The language on the page also does not inspire confidence, referring to "Y sperms" and "X sperms" (*sperm* is already plural, dude).

You don't need to buy a $439 kit to use at-home sex-selection methods. Follow the timing recommendations, take some calcium (girl) or potassium (boy) supplements, eat lots of food if you want a boy, and . . . pray. Most important of all, remember: No matter what the gender of your child, he or she will be a joy.

CHAPTER 6

Not as Scary as You've Heard: The Real Stats on Age and Fertility

You've probably heard lots of scary statistics on getting pregnant in your 30s, particularly after age 35. Not long ago, doctors used terms such as "advanced geriatric status," "senile gravida," and "elderly prima gravida" to describe pregnant women over 35, as if 35-year-old women regularly hobbled into their offices using walkers, their support hose bunching around their wrinkled ankles. I was 34 when I tried to get pregnant for the first time, and we knew we wanted at least two children and didn't want them just a year apart. So I tried to find out how hard it would be to get pregnant after 35.

The statistic I saw most often—on numerous websites and in books—said that only two out of three 35-year-old women would be pregnant after a year of unprotected sex. That meant one out of three wouldn't, and no pregnancy after a year is a common definition for infertility. When you really want to have a baby, facing a one in three shot of being infertile is downright frightening.

But I was curious—where did this statistic come from? I found the citation to the original research, published in the medical journal *Human Reproduction*, and read the article. When I got to the part where the author described his data, I laughed out loud—not my usual reaction to dry medical articles. The data, it turns out, were from church birth records in rural France between 1670 and 1830! Surely some of those older women who already had seven or more children were able to fend off their husbands occasionally? And didn't the French discover withdrawal right around then? Not to mention that life expectancy was much shorter, and modern medicine, antibiotics, and indoor plumbing didn't exist. Did they even have soap? This is a very different situation from the healthy modern woman who wants to get pregnant and lures her husband into bed with the siren song, "I'm ovulating!" Healthy lifestyles can't completely trump biological aging, of course, but surely these groups had some key differences from our situations now—timing sex based on ovulation being the most obvious.

But these and similar statistics are everywhere. The American Society for Reproductive Medicine put out a booklet saying that 30 percent of women who started trying to get pregnant between the ages of 35 and 39 would never have a child, citing another study of 350-year-old birth records. The booklet also says that the chance of getting pregnant per cycle is 20 percent for a 30-year-old but only 5 percent per cycle for a 40-year-old, a widely reported statistic contradicted by several research studies (see Chapter 1).

There had to be better data. I soon found it, and it was much more encouraging. A study in the 1990s of couples

having sex at least twice a week found that 50 percent of 35-
to 39-year-old women were pregnant after three months,
and 82 percent were pregnant within a year. (If you've been
trying for more than three months, don't assume that there
must be something wrong. These numbers are the average,
so half of couples will take longer.) The study also found
that many couples who didn't get pregnant in the first year
got pregnant in the second year of trying naturally; at the
end of two years, 90 percent of 35- to 39-year-old women
were pregnant. Sex two days before ovulation led to pregnancy among 25 percent of 35- to 39-year-old women after
just one cycle—the same percentage of women aged 19 to
26 who got pregnant when they had sex three days before
ovulation. So timing sex just one day better eliminated the
age difference in fertility. If you follow the recommendations in this book, you might be able to get pregnant just as
quickly as someone a decade younger.

What if you're approaching 30? Is it better to get started
right now, since (as so many websites like to point out) fertility starts to drop around age 27? Not really. The study
found no noticeable difference in fertility for couples in
their early 30s compared to those in their late 20s.

Of course, there are notable age-related declines in fertility. An incredible 50 percent of women aged 19 to 26 in
this study got pregnant when they had sex two days before
ovulation (hopefully not from the condom breaking!), compared to 25 percent of the 35-to-39-year-olds. It's easy to
spin this the scary way: Breaking News: Fertility Cut in Half
When You're Over 35!! But a one in four chance of getting pregnant from just one roll in the hay isn't bad when

your 20th high school reunion is fast approaching—or even over. The bottom line: Most 35- to 39-year-old women will be able to get pregnant naturally, but it might take a few months longer than for younger women.

The Fifth Decade

What about fertility after 40? I couldn't find any modern studies on natural conception after 40 (which is appalling, really, given the interest in this topic). The historical birth records show that 44 percent of 40-year-old women got pregnant in a year, and 64 percent within 4 years. The average woman had her last child at age 41. But I'm not sure those numbers would apply today in the age of fertility monitors, better health, and not already being the mother of eight.

The only modern statistics come from fertility treatments. Per IVF cycle, 50 percent of those under 35 go home with a baby, compared to 30 percent at 35 to 39, 14 percent at 40, 8 to 10 percent at 41 to 43, and 2 to 3 percent at 44 to 45. (Realize these statistics are for *one* cycle, and many couples try more than once.) Some of this decline is due to aging eggs, which also affects natural conception. But the drop is also due to the mechanics of IVF, which work best if the ovaries produce a lot of eggs at once. That's less likely to happen if you're older. For natural conception, though, all it takes is one.

If you're 40 or older, some doctors advise trying on your own for only three months before seeing a fertility specialist. This advice is based on the idea that you should pursue treatment sooner rather than later to increase your odds of success. If you can afford it, ruling out any tubal or sperm issues right away is a great idea. But if those tests are normal, your best chance for a baby might be from natural conception, because the IVF process favors younger women. If you're over 40, ovulation prediction using the methods in Chapter 3 can help you make the most of the chances you have left. You never know which month will have your lucky, normal egg, and if you hit all of them, you have a much better chance of success. Following the other recommendations in this book, such as taking prenatal vitamins and getting rid of bad habits, can also increase your chances.

When Carey Goldberg, coauthor of the fertility memoir *Three Wishes*, was 39 (an age she describes as "biological midnight"), she chose a sperm donor and bought three vials of sperm. She then met a man named Sprax (no, that's not a typo) on an online dating site. He agreed to be her "natural sperm donor"—he wasn't sure he wanted to be a husband and father. Carey suffered a miscarriage a week after her 40th birthday, but then, with the help of a fertility monitor, went on to have a healthy pregnancy and a beautiful baby girl when she was 41. Two years later, at 43, she had a baby boy. Eventually, she and Sprax even became a solid couple and got married. Carey passed on the unused vials of donor sperm to two of her friends, both of whom went on to have children at 41, and with real-life men instead of the donor sperm (though not without problems along the way). It's a great story of love, struggle, and ultimately the joy of over-40 motherhood.

Miscarriage and Birth Defects

Of course, there are downsides to getting pregnant after 35. Miscarriages are more common: About 10 percent of pregnancies miscarry among women under 30, about 12 percent for those 30 to 34, 18 percent for those 35 to 39, and 34 percent for those 40 to 44. However, the majority of pregnancies, even for women in their 40s, will be fine. Most of the time, miscarriages are caused by chromosomal mistakes in the embryo. This happens more often in older women because their eggs have more abnormalities. But women aren't alone in feeling the effects of age on fertility. The man's age also plays a role in miscarriages and in chromosomal birth defects such as Down syndrome. When you have a miscarriage, though, it doesn't matter whose fault it is, and neither one of you can make yourselves younger. So you just have to try again. The good news is you're very likely to carry a pregnancy to term the next time. (See Chapter 9 for more about miscarriage.)

You might have heard that it's dangerous for women over 35 to have children due to the risk of birth defects. That's just not true. Although the rate of birth defects does rise as women age, the risk is still very, very low. Among 35-year-old women, 99.5 percent of babies will be chromosomally normal at delivery, and 0.5 percent, or 1 in 204, will not be. Among 40-year-old women, 98.5 percent of babies will be chromosomally normal, and 1.5 percent, or 1 in 65, will not be. At 45, when very few women can still get pregnant, 95 percent of babies will still be chromosomally normal, and 5 percent (1 in 20) will not be. (These numbers are a little higher at early genetic testing, probably because abnormal fetuses are more likely to miscarry or be stillborn.) Interestingly, the majority of Down syndrome babies are born to women younger than 35. (Their risk is lower, but they have more babies.)

If even these small risks seem daunting, several prenatal screening tests are available. A special ultrasound (called nucheal translucency) can detect about 80 percent of cases of Down's in the first trimester, and there's no risk of miscarriage from the procedure. This test is often combined with blood tests in the first and second trimesters (called sequential screening). Other tests, such as amniocentesis and chorionic villus sampling (CVS), can detect Down's and other chromosomal problems with 99 percent accuracy. Both amnio and CVS carry a small risk of miscarriage—about half a percent. The advantage of CVS is that it can be done earlier, around 11 weeks. I had CVS in each of my three pregnancies and was able to learn at less than three months along that I was carrying a chromosomally normal baby.

Tests for Fertility in Older Women

If you're older than 30, you've probably wondered if you're less fertile and how much time you have left to have the family you want. Several at-home tests have emerged to try to answer that question. Unfortunately, the information they give you might be less than helpful.

The First Response Fertility Test comes in a pink box that asks, "Are you able to get pregnant?" The problem is that a test in a box is not going to be able to answer that question—it can't, for example, see if your fallopian tubes are open. The test measures the level of follicle-stimulating hormone (FSH), which is higher in women approaching menopause. The First Response test doesn't tell you a number for your FSH level, as a doctor's office test would—it just turns positive or negative. If it's like most at-home FSH tests, it turns positive around 25 mIU/ml, a level that most women wouldn't get unless they were already experiencing the symptoms of menopause. So the test doesn't really give you much useful information. Other home FSH tests turn positive at 10 mIU/ml, a common cutoff for "high FSH." Yet many studies find that FSH at this level doesn't predict fertility very well. My friend Kendall is the ultimate proof of this: She got pregnant with her third child—naturally—at the age of 40, the same cycle a blood test showed her FSH was 25.

Another test, called Plan Ahead, requires a blood test and measures other markers (such as anti-Müllerian hormone, or AMH) along with FSH. The manufacturers call this a test of "ovarian reserve" or "remaining egg supply" and say it will tell you how many years of fertility you have left. It gives you a specific number ranging between 1 and 30, a rough indication of the number of antral follicles in your ovaries—the fewer you have, the closer you presumably are to menopause. A fertility doctor can also do an ultrasound and count your antral follicles. An antral follicle count of 10 or less—the average for a woman in her early 40s—is called *diminished ovarian reserve*. Some fertility doctors are very ominous about ovarian reserve, noting that this is one of the few fertility problems modern medicine has found almost impossible to treat.

Should all 30-year-old women who have not yet had their last child have one of these tests, as some experts have suggested? Probably not, because having a low ovarian reserve doesn't mean you can't get pregnant—it just means the hyperstimulation of the ovaries required for IVF doesn't work very well. Studies of women conceiving naturally find that ovarian reserve doesn't predict who gets pregnant and who doesn't. As British gynecologist Dimitrios Nikolaou says, "Ovarian reserve tests should be relabeled ovarian response tests." (Ovarian response means how many eggs doctors can get out during IVF.) The website of the Advanced Fertility Center of Chicago comes to a similar conclusion: "The quantity of remaining eggs probably does not have a large impact on natural fertility. However, when going through a fertility treatment such as IVF, the quantity of eggs remaining influences response to ovarian-stimulating medications." So these tests can't really predict your chances of getting pregnant naturally.

I took the Plan Ahead test in 2008, before we were going to start trying for a second child and before I knew about the limited utility of these tests. My result was an 8, well below average for someone my age (37 at the time). A few months later, an ultrasound showed I had only 5 antral follicles. I found a website that gave the antral follicle count and the number of years until the woman had her last child. Next to 5 there was a dash—that is, those women didn't have any more children. Between crying jags, I wondered if we would ever have a second child. As it turned out, I got a positive pregnancy test the next day, and my second daughter was born nine months later. More than two years later, when I was almost 40 and presumably had even fewer eggs, I got pregnant in just two months of trying. Maybe I should email my children's pictures to the website.

The Psychology of Age and Fertility

Age is a frustrating aspect of fertility because you can't change it, and it just keeps getting worse as the days go by. Women are already sensitive about age in our youth-centered, Botoxed society. Worries about fertility just add another layer of anxiety to something we can't do anything about. The good news is you are probably better prepared for pregnancy and parenthood now than when you were younger. You're also more likely to have the financial resources to eat better, exercise, and take care of yourself. Commenting on the press coverage about age and fertility in 2001, Tina Fey remarked on *Saturday Night Live*, "According to author Sylvia Hewlett, career women shouldn't wait to have babies because our fertility takes a steep drop-off after age 27. And Sylvia's right; I *definitely* should have had a baby when I was 27, living in Chicago over a biker bar, pulling down a cool $12,000 a year. That would have worked out great."

Some of us are childless at 35 or older because relationships didn't go the way we'd hoped. We might have gotten divorced, devoted years to a man who wouldn't commit, or just not found our mate until later. Carey Goldberg, the

Three Wishes author, was a foreign correspondent until she was 34. She returned to the United States with, she says, "the very explicit idea of Getting a Life." But that turned out to be more difficult than she had hoped. "What I want most in life now is to fall in love, marry, and have a family, but that is not the sort of thing you can make happen," she told a friend at the time. "You can't go to school for it. You can't get on a waiting list for it. You can't directly apply. You can try to prepare for it, but what else?"

Whatever you do, don't blame yourself. What's past is past, and you have to accept the age you are. It's very easy to get panicked about things you read about age and fertility, and so much of what's out there is slanted in one way or another because that makes a better headline. For some reason, everyone loves to begin their article with the scary line, "Women are born with all the eggs they will ever have." (Which always makes me want to scream. I was born with all of the arms I will ever have, too, and they're working just fine, thank you.)

Magazine and newspaper stories often rely on questionable statistics or, when they have correct statistics, spin them in a way that sounds terrifying. When I was 30 and had not yet met my husband, I read a *Newsweek* cover article that began by noting that only 2 percent of babies are born to mothers 40 or over. That makes it sound as if a 40-year-old woman has only a 2 percent chance of having a baby, which isn't even close to true. The reason so few babies are born to mothers over 40 is that most 40-year-old women aren't trying to get pregnant—usually because they've had their children already. So that's a very misleading statistic.

Once again, the women of *Saturday Night Live* nailed

it. Tina Fey cracked, "The cover story of *New York Magazine* this week is 'Baby Panic.' This goes perfectly with the other magazines on my coffee table: 'Where Are the Babies?' *(Us)*, 'Why Haven't You Had a Baby?' *(People)*, and 'For God's Sake Have a Baby' *(Time)*. Thanks, *Time* magazine. This is just what I need—another article *so* depressing that I can actually hear my ovaries curling up." Rachel Dratch followed that with, "Yeah, thanks for reminding me that I have to hurry up and have a baby. Uh, me and my four cats will get *right* on that." Amy Poehler said, "My neighbor has this adorable, cute little Chinese baby that speaks Italian. So, you know, I'll just buy one of those." The fun coda to this riff is that Tina Fey had her second child at 40, Rachel Dratch got pregnant (apparently accidentally) at 43, and Amy Poehler had her second child at 38. Much of America witnessed Amy's first pregnancy during the 2008 election season, when she bounced around the studio doing her Sarah Palin rap while a huge nine months pregnant. She had her first son just a week later, at the age of 37.

Even research articles in otherwise staid and boring medical journals manage to make age and fertility emotionally charged. My favorite, written by three men, noted that "many women have elected to postpone their first pregnancy until after age 35" (as if this was an arbitrary and completely voluntary choice) and thus, "unfortunately, a substantial proportion of these women will be unable to conceive naturally due to the corrosive effects of age." (I bet age had a "corrosive effect" on your wrinkled butt, too, buddy). They then complain that "many women do not realize" the effect of age on fertility, as if this hadn't been beaten into our heads since puberty. They ominously conclude that "with each birthday come reductions in follicular [egg] numbers." Just think about *that* at your next birthday party! Have fun! At least we're not getting more annoying with each birthday like these guys.

What's the Deadline?

If you have a demanding career, like to travel, want your children to be several years apart, or want to enjoy more years of childless freedom, you've probably wondered how long you can wait to try to get pregnant. You might have heard the scary statistics trumpeting that fertility starts to decline at 27. It does, but not by much. After 35, and especially after 40, the decline in fertility becomes more steep, and after 45 pregnancy is rare. You've probably heard stories of women who had children well into their 40s or even know a woman who did. My aunt was nearly 43 when she had my cousin, her first and only child. My great-aunt Francie had her ninth child at 43, and then—incredibly—another at 48. (This was in the 1940s, with no fertility treatment involved.) But we remember these stories precisely because they are so unusual. When you read about celebrities who had children in their late 40s or early 50s, they almost always used donor eggs.

If you want more than one child, you'll have to do what I call "woman math." How many children do you want, and how many years apart would you like to space them? For a sample woman math equation, imagine you want to have three children two years apart by the time you are 37. You'll want to have the first at 33, with the second coming at 35, and the last at 37. It's usually better for your physical and mental health for children to be at least two years apart, but if you're pushing 40 or over, you might not be able to allow that much time. I had my first two children three years apart and wished I could have spaced them even further. It's easier if you can get your older one potty trained and in a big bed by the time you have a newborn, and we missed by a few months on both counts. We got two years and three months between our second and third, which was adequate but not ideal. If you plan on breastfeeding, realize you won't be at top fertility until after you wean the baby, which could be at a year or even two. Some women want to have all of their children by the time they are 35, thinking that risks for Down syndrome go up after that age, but that's not how it works—the risk increases steadily as you age, and there's nothing magic about age 35.

It's true that having your children when you are younger has numerous benefits. You're likely to get pregnant faster and will be less likely to miscarry, and you'll have more energy for chasing young kids around. But the chances are still very good that you will have no problem getting pregnant and carrying a baby up until your late 30s and even very early 40s. If you're wondering how much time you have, the frustrating thing is there is no way to tell for sure. Each woman has to make the decision for herself about how long is too long to wait and how old is too old. The good news is the statistics aren't as scary as they're often made out to be—unless you're a woman in 17th-century France. Isn't it awesome that we're not?

"If One More Person Tells Me to 'Just Relax' . . .": The Psychological Side of Getting Pregnant

The stories of infertile couples are everywhere—online, in books, and spread from friend to friend. Everyone is afraid they will be next. Even without any real reason to expect a problem, I worried endlessly that I wouldn't be able to get pregnant, as did many women I know.

Even though the vast majority of women won't have a fertility problem, any possibility of not being able to have a baby can be anxiety provoking. It's a roller coaster of emotions over the course of a month: waiting to try, trying, waiting to see if it worked, and finding out it didn't. Then you start over the next month. Once you've been trying for three months, six months, or a year, and nothing is happening, it can send you over the edge. "It takes you over, mind, body, and soul," said Beth when she'd been trying to conceive her second child for six months. (It took another year of trying, but she finally got pregnant and had a healthy baby girl.)

Marie and her husband tried to get pregnant for four

and a half years before finally succeeding with their first try at IVF. When I asked her how she managed not to fall apart (I would have been certifiably insane after six months), she said, "You get through it. You go on because you have no other choice." I tried to remember this when I would feel my heart plummet into my stomach after getting my period. Even though we'd only been trying for a few months, I couldn't imagine waiting even one more month. Unfortunately, knowing that other women had it worse didn't help me feel better. I just felt bad for them, too.

Many people will tell you that you'll get pregnant if you "stop trying" or "just relax," which is ridiculous. It would be a lot more relaxing if people would stop telling us to "just relax," because then we wouldn't have to fight the urge to smack them. Fortunately, worrying about trying to get pregnant will not make you infertile. If you worry so much for so long that you become depressed, though, that can affect fertility (see Chapter 1).

Why Trying to Get Pregnant Is So Anxiety Provoking

I spent my late 20s in a basement in Cleveland, rejecting people. I'd taken a job as a researcher at Case Western Reserve University, working in the lab of an eminent social psychologist. We developed a research program to study what happens when people are socially rejected by others. I'd get a group of college students together, have them talk for 15 minutes, separate them, and ask them to choose who they wanted to pair up with for the next activity. Then I'd tell half of them that no one chose them. The other, luckier half would hear that everyone chose them. Over the course of a dozen experiments, we found that the rejected students procrastinated more, ate more cookies, made more risky choices, thought time was passing slowly, were more aggressive, and were less willing to help other people. Getting rejected by a few people they met for only 15 minutes really messed them up.

We are hardwired to need other people and to want to create relationships. If rejection from a group of strangers hurts, it makes a lot of sense that fertility—which creates a bond with a child, one of the most important relationships in life—provokes deep-seated feelings of anxiety. Throw in the strong biological drive to reproduce, the comforting thought that your children are likely to outlive you, and the sense of purpose people get from parenting, and you have a perfect storm of human desires: companionship, reproduction, fear of death, meaning in life. Trying to get pregnant pushes so many of our psychological buttons at once. If you are going crazy, there are some very good reasons for that, and it's not just you.

But that doesn't mean it feels good—in fact, it feels awful. Here are some strategies to keep the crazy at bay.

Ways to Cope

⟿ **Take action.** Read books like this one, gather information, buy a fertility monitor, and have sex. The key is finding a balance. Try not to obsess so much that you drive yourself (or your husband) crazy. And after a point, you are probably doing everything you can. After ovulation, you can't really do anything, so you have to stop researching cervical mucus and start researching how to calm the heck down. This is one of the keys to coping: Actively focus on what you can change and let go of what you can't.

↪ **Stop ruminating.** For many women, taking in information can easily turn into thinking about fertility all the time. Your mind wanders there whenever you have a free moment, and you're turning it over and over in your head when you're exercising, doing a boring task at work, watching TV, or making dinner. Psychologists call this rumination, and it's a strong predictor for developing serious depression. (Yeah, I know: Now you're anxious about your anxiety. D'oh! But read on.) Women are particularly prone to ruminate—it's one of the main reasons twice as many women as men become depressed. Somehow guys have mastered the art of chilling out and watching the game on TV instead of thinking all the time. Lucky bastards. So the first step is to act like a guy. Recognize when you start ruminating, stop it, and do something else. Don't try to convince yourself that ruminating on and off for hours is helping you solve your problem. Tell yourself you can think about a problem for 10 minutes (because any good ideas will come in the first 10 minutes anyway) and then stop.

It's usually easiest to stop ruminating if you can do something more active that fully involves your mind. One of the best ways is distraction: Do something else, preferably something that requires your complete attention so that your mind won't wander. (For more on this, see Susan

Nolen-Hoeksema's book *Women Who Think Too Much*. Isn't that all of us?) Do something you really enjoy, like reading a good book, doing art projects, working on sudoku or crossword puzzles, shopping, gardening, hiking, or exercising. Just make sure it's engaging enough that your mind won't wander. I love to swim for exercise, but I found myself ruminating about fertility a lot when I was swimming. I still swam—exercise is a great natural mood booster—but I tried to actively think about something else. And the rest of the time I distracted myself by doing more engaging things like reading a page-turner novel or watching a movie.

↬ **Write in a journal.** A series of amazing research studies find that if you write about stressful things, your mental and physical health improve. This was true even if people threw away what they wrote and didn't expect anyone to ever read it. Somehow putting the words and emotions on paper released these feelings. It sounds similar to rumination—aren't you mulling over the same things?—but once it's put on paper (or into a computer file), it stops rolling around in your head over and over. You're less likely to cover the same ground and more likely to feel a release. You don't have to write in a formal journal, and you don't have to write every day or even every week—just write when you're upset or anxious, on scrap paper or on your laptop.

↬ **Show gratitude.** When you're writing in your journal, don't just write about the negative stuff. Start by listing 5 to 10 things you are grateful for: your husband, your friends, your job, your house, even little things like the warmth of the sunlight or the snuggle of your flannel sheets. People who are grateful for what they already have are happier, and it's easy to see why: They're thinking about how to enjoy what's in front of them instead of focusing on what's still out of reach. Showing gratitude can be difficult when it feels like all you want is a baby, but taking the time to appreciate your blessings will lift your mood.

↬ **Find natural mood boosters.** Dr. Steve Ilardi of the University of Kansas has done some remarkable research showing that changes in lifestyle can alleviate depression just as well as medication (see his excellent book *The Depression Cure*). Even better, these strategies can reduce anxiety and prevent depression. His advice overlaps with many of the lifestyle suggestions earlier in this book. The six steps are:

1. Avoid rumination (catch yourself when you're mulling over your problems and stop).
2. Get out in natural sunlight (at least 15 to 30 minutes a day, ideally in the morning; some people use a light box).
3. Take an omega-3 supplement with at least 1,000 milligrams of EPA.
4. Exercise regularly (at least 90 minutes a week).
5. Get enough sleep (at least 8 hours a night).
6. Spend time with friends and family.

These steps sound simple, but they are exactly the things most of us lack in the modern world. You might not be able to realistically do all of them. But you can try, and more than likely they will help. Dr. Ilardi reports lasting effects in his patients, and, unlike with drugs, there are no side effects.

Exercise can also be used as a short-term fix. Pounding

the pavement, chopping through the water, or hitting the pedals is virtually guaranteed to take the edge off your anxiety and sadness. And maybe you'll even get a great butt.

↬ **Try relaxation techniques.** Some of the anxiety around trying to conceive is chronic—it drags on and on for months. Other times, the anxiety arrives all at once in the wildly beating heart and fast breathing that can border on a panic attack. This can happen when you're taking your temperature in the morning, using the fertility monitor, taking a pregnancy test, checking the toilet paper near the end of your cycle, or waiting for a phone call about blood test results. To prepare for these moments, take a few minutes now—when you are hopefully *not* anxious—to learn the technique of deep breathing. Close your eyes and concentrate on taking slow, deep breaths until you feel your body relax. Some people also imagine a relaxing place, such as a quiet beach or a forest. One way to practice is to tense and then release different muscles in your body so that you learn how to voluntarily relax. If you practice in advance, it's easier to employ these techniques when your brain is telling you to freak out. The idea is to relax your body so that your mind will eventually follow. The technique is very similar to yoga or meditation, so if you've done one of those, you know the basics already.

Once you learn deep breathing, it's useful in all kinds of situations—for example, it's the same method women use in natural childbirth. It's also useful when you're at work trying not to blow up at an annoying coworker or at home when your husband asks where the wine opener is when you've told him 20 times before. Anytime you feel yourself getting upset or anxious, try to breathe deeply and relax. You'll send the signal to your body that everything is fine and you will feel less panicky. Some people call these brief deep breathing episodes "minis" (or, as one IW misremembered it, "quickies"—she got the connection to fertility, but just in a different area!). Minis are useful for all of those times when you think you're going to lose it, like hearing a friend is pregnant or waiting for the results of a pregnancy test.

One variation on this technique is Tonglen meditation, created in the mountains of Tibet. To perform Tonglen, you have to accept your anxiety or pain and imagine breathing it in. Then you exhale it out, slowly, thinking of peace and relaxation. Tonglen is more difficult because it requires embracing your fear, but it can be more cleansing because it involves accepting and then expelling your negative feelings instead of just trying to relax them away.

Perhaps you already have a favorite way to relax, like getting a massage, going to yoga class, using aromatherapy, or getting acupuncture. If these help you, you'll definitely want to continue doing them while you're trying to get pregnant, and probably do them more. And if you've never tried massage or yoga, this might be just the time to indulge. Warm baths and hot tubs are also great ways to relax (though you'll want to avoid water over 100°F after you get a positive pregnancy test). Jackie, who battled infertility for two years, swore by Epsom salt baths. She says they not only relaxed her but gave her what felt like a runner's high, but without the annoying running!

↪ **Challenge negative thoughts.** Psychologist Dr. Alice

Domar has published a series of remarkable studies showing that infertile women felt better and were more likely to get pregnant after participating in cognitive-behavioral therapy. These women practiced the relaxation techniques previously mentioned and learned how to challenge their negative thoughts, rephrasing them to be more positive. For example, one woman kept thinking, "I will never have a baby." She learned to shift that thought to "I am doing everything I can to try to get pregnant." You'll notice that this technique doesn't just rely on the empty "positive thinking" promoted by pop psychology, which would instead suggest thinking something like, "I know I will have a baby," which could lead to disappointment. In *Conquering Infertility*, Dr. Domar suggests women remember, "You will be happy again. Life will become joyful again. And somehow, some way, if you want to become a parent, you will."

If you're feeling down but think you're not depressed, therapy might still be a good idea. Very often, depressed people don't want to admit that they are depressed. You might think you will be able to snap out of it in a few weeks or when you're pregnant. When that doesn't happen, it just makes you feel worse, which makes it even less likely you'll get pregnant. The symptoms of depression aren't necessarily the things you'd think; they include changes in sleep patterns, difficulty thinking of anything other than fertility, and diminished ability to accomplish tasks.

⤙ **Seek group support.** Dr. Domar's research also found good results when women joined in-person support groups in which they shared developments and talked about relationships. Group leaders addressed the impact of infertility on work, spirituality, family, and other areas. If you're interested in joining a support group, the infertility group Resolve is a great place to start.

If you're not at the stage where you want to join a group, you can still talk to people you know. Mothers, sisters, and friends can be great listeners. Sometimes, though, they aren't, and they say insensitive yet well-intentioned things. ("Just relax and it will happen." "Don't worry about it because it's out of your control." "If it's meant to be, it will happen.") If you're just starting trying to get pregnant, these comments won't bother you much and you'll probably still benefit from talking to someone you love and trust. But if you've been trying for more than six months (the point at which many women get frustrated), or had an early loss or a miscarriage, my advice is to talk to someone who has been through these experiences. They know through hard-won experience that just relaxing doesn't fix everything. When I had an early miscarriage, I called two friends: one who had experienced a miscarriage and another who'd fought infertility for years before having her daughter. They told me it would get better every day, which it did. In short, they talked me off the wall and I am forever grateful.

And know this simple fact: If struggling to get pregnant has made you feel crazy, you are not alone. Dr. Domar found that infertility patients were just as depressed as *cancer* patients. Struggling to get pregnant is apparently just as depressing as facing down a deadly disease. If you feel this way, you are responding the way many women do, and it is not your fault. But just because it's common doesn't mean it's acceptable. Join a support group or get therapy.

You will be happier, and you might even be more likely to get pregnant.

⇨ **Use online message boards.** An easy, always available form of group support is online message boards, which can connect you with other women who are going through the same experience (whether that's TTC naturally, infertility treatment, miscarriage, or any other situation). They can be fantastic support in many cases, especially if you don't know anyone in real life who's TTC, or don't want to talk about TTC with anyone you actually know. Some women love boards and some hate them (or love some boards and hate others—shop around if you don't find one you like right away).

Don't expect message boards to take the place of your in-person relationships. Online relationships are anonymous and accessible, and you can connect with many people who have had similar experiences—something that can be hard to do in real life. The downside is you lose nuance when interacting online, and the anonymity can sometimes feel empty. Message boards can lead to anxiety if you post something and no one responds—or, worse, other posters say something unhelpful or even insulting. Online interactions can become contentious very quickly if someone has a strong opinion. Even when others are being supportive, message boards can sometimes become one big collective rumination fest, with women going over and over the same problems. You have to know when to walk away.

Reading about someone else's problems can sometimes make you feel worse. You're glad you're not alone, but feel sad for them as well as for yourself. You lose the context of an in-person relationship where you might know more about the other person and can see they can still smile. Because people are most likely to post on the boards when they are having trouble or feeling down, the boards can make things look scarier than they actually are. Then there's the opposite problem—woman after woman announcing her BFP (big fat positive) on her pregnancy test as you stay there still trying to conceive month after month. Then you peek over at the boards for infertility, and all of the doctors' appointments and procedures seem so scary. As Tiffany told me, "Sometimes those postings gave me more anxiety than comfort."

The advice you get on message boards runs the gamut. It can be fantastic—many women who chart their cycles or use a fertility monitor first heard about these things on message boards. But more precise pieces of advice are harder to come by. (Have you seen some of the completely idiotic things people post on Yahoo! Answers?) Reading the boards for advice is fine, but do so with the realization that not everything you read will be right, and you'll have to look into it further to separate the myths from the truths. It's always hard to say whether the magic technique or supplement someone raves about had anything to do with her getting pregnant. It could have just been her lucky cycle. This goes for the advice of people you know in real life as well. It's so easy to believe something will work for you because it worked for someone else. When I saw something on a message board or even in a book, I'd research it to see if there had been any studies showing it actually worked. Sometimes there was evidence it did, but more often studies showed it didn't work. More often than not, there were no studies at all—probably why there is so much speculation on message boards.

↬ **Consider defensive pessimism.** You've probably heard that being optimistic is always best. Expect the best to happen, the thinking goes, and it will. That's good advice when your actions have direct consequences. But for something partially out of your control like getting pregnant, being optimistic can sometimes really mess you up. Let's say you are optimistic and expect to get pregnant the first cycle you try. If you do, your expectations are fulfilled. If you don't, you're really disappointed (and even more disappointed if it still hasn't happened after six months). If you are less optimistic, even a little pessimistic, you tell yourself it's unlikely that you'll get pregnant on the first try and that it will probably take about six months. Then if you get pregnant on your first try, you're pleasantly surprised. If you don't, it's what you expected.

This viewpoint is called defensive pessimism. (For more on it, read *The Positive Power of Negative Thinking* by Julie Norem.) Defensive pessimism is *not* thinking that drags you into depression (such as "I'll never get pregnant"; "It's been three months, so there must be something wrong with me"). Instead, it's a strategy of preparing yourself for negative outcomes before they happen and setting your expectations at a low to medium level so that you're not too disappointed. I realize I already undermined this approach by giving you those very positive statistics about time to pregnancy in Chapter 1 and again in Chapter 6. But defensive pessimism is more about perception than statistics—

it's about protecting yourself from getting your hopes up too high.

The year I turned 30, I embarked on a whirlwind of dating. I soon found that the potential for disappointment was huge. Someone who was really funny and nice online just wouldn't have that spark in person. Someone who seemed okay online would turn out to be absolutely horrible in person. One Wednesday a friend asked me what I was doing that night, and I muttered dejectedly, "I have another date." The guy had sounded nice on the phone, but his profile picture was blurry—it looked like his work badge. I was expecting another disaster. But when I arrived at the restaurant, I almost did a double take at the man who said my name. He was so cute! We hit it off right away, and—as you've probably guessed by now—he became my husband two years later. I lost nothing by going into the date with low expectations, but protected myself in case I was disappointed. (And yes, the blurry photo was his work badge.)

The same strategy can work well for getting pregnant. Each cycle is like an Internet date: It's got a chance of working out but also a chance of going down in flames. You should still do what you can to help it go well—time sex right, take your vitamins—but if it doesn't work, that's what you expected. Online, I came across a blogger who did what she called "perfunctory IUI #7" in between IVF tries. After the procedure, she wrote, "It has opened up a whole new world of freedom. I expect nothing from this cycle, and therefore I cannot be disappointed." As it turned out, that was the cycle she conceived twins after seven years of infertility, eventually delivering a healthy boy and girl. Defensive pessimism allows you to protect yourself, but it still allows for joy when things work out.

 ➴ **Use humor.** It's okay to laugh about infertility—and it might help you feel better, or even help you get pregnant. Among women undergoing IVF, those who were entertained by a clown right after the embryo transfer were twice as likely to get pregnant. That's presumably because the clown helped them laugh a little (or scared them enough to get them good and pregnant—but then, I'm in the camp that thinks clowns are a little frightening). The study researcher hopes there will be more research on clowns and fertility: "After all," he said, "this is one of the least hazardous interventions in our field." He's probably right that clowns are less scary than a hypodermic filled with progesterone. Well, maybe.

Humor won't be the first thing that occurs to you when you're sad, but it's a great diversion when you're anxious. Watch a funny movie that has nothing to do with fertility, or watch one that has everything to do with it. (*Baby Mama* is a good one.) Or read a fertility humor book—yes, they exist! (For example, check out *The Conception Chronicles.*) Or make jokes yourself; dark humor is a great coping mechanism. Try to see the ridiculous in the things that make you anxious. Sometimes this is easy. OPK and pregnancy test sticks are inherently funny because they involve pee (the root of all elementary school humor), and baby-making is inherently funny because it involves sex (the root of all adolescent humor). All of it is more fun than being an actual adult.

⮕ **Consider faith and spirituality.** Faith can be a safe refuge during many times in life, but it is especially helpful when facing difficult, uncontrollable circumstances—and struggling to get pregnant certainly qualifies. Many people believe that God has a plan for them. This belief can be a great comfort because it imbues everything with meaning and lets you know that it will be okay in the end. If you need infertility treatment, perhaps you will cherish your children even more or help others who are going through the same experience. If you end up adopting, perhaps you will feel you were meant to parent that child. Nicole, 30, was trying to conceive for a year, got pregnant, and then miscarried. Her faith helped her get through a very difficult time. "The miscarriage was one of my biggest fears, and God had me face it head on—on Mother's Day weekend!" she wrote. "But I was overwhelmed by the peace that God had a bigger plan for us. It washed over me and carried me through. I know that God knows the desire of my heart and that He will guide us in this process."

It can be difficult, though, if you really want a baby and wonder if God is punishing you, or if you feel angry at God. Carrie, 37, says that when she was trying to get pregnant and got her period, "I would get really mad at God." These feelings are common, but they can be very destructive to your faith and to your mental health. Try to talk them through with a therapist or your religious leader. And when you have doubts, or wonder if you're being punished, realize that God does not expect you to be perfect. Ask for forgiveness from God or from whomever you wronged. Forgiveness lightens the soul and begins the journey to healing. As one woman on a fertility message board wrote in her signature, "God will never give me more than I can handle. I just wish He didn't trust me so much!" The rest of her signature was two beautiful and highly relevant Bible verses: (1) "Don't worry about anything; instead, pray about everything." (2) "When you go through deep waters and great trouble, I will be with you."

⤙ **Limit your exposure.** When you first start trying to conceive or are thinking about it, talking to pregnant women or women with babies is really fun. You ask them about their experience, joyfully thinking that this will be you soon. But that joy can quickly turn to jealousy when you have a hard time getting pregnant. Friends call to announce their pregnancies and you have to try to be happy for them. Invitations for baby showers and birthday parties make you want to cry. Everywhere you look, there are reminders that other people have what you want so much. As my friend Beth wrote, "It hurts to see a mother holding her infant, see the tiny diapers of a newborn, see a big, round belly. It hurts to long with every fiber of my being for a baby and not know if I will have one."

It is fine to send a gift and avoid the baby shower, and fine to politely change the subject when yet another person asks if you're ever going to have kids. Jessica, 31, says, "I've had to 'hide' many friends and a few family members on Facebook due to their many pregnancy updates. I just couldn't face that day after day. I've also scheduled appointments to coincide with baby shower events as a cop-out, passing along a gift at another time."

Try not to shut out too many people for too long. When

you do get pregnant, you will want those friendships with women who have children. And, fortunately, most people will be very supportive.

↬ **Ask about antidepressant medication.** One out of nine Americans took antidepressant medication (such as Prozac, Paxil, or Wellbutrin) in 2008, twice the rate as in the 1990s. You might be one of them or you might be considering it. Recent research shows that antidepressants don't work very well for mild depression, but they produce meaningful improvements for people who are severely depressed. If you're feeling anxious and wonder how long you'll be able to hold things together, try the other strategies in this chapter first before going on medication. You'll avoid the side effects and won't have to worry about changing or going off the meds when you're pregnant. But if you're still feeling bad—particularly if your anxiety has crashed into serious depression—antidepressants may very well be the best choice. Talk to your doctor about which antidepressants are safe when you're trying to conceive or are pregnant.

Fertility and Your Relationship with Your Partner

At first, trying to get pregnant is great for your relationship—the shared promise, the feeling you're creating something together, the excuse to have more sex. If you have trouble getting pregnant or even worry about having trouble, all of that fun comes to a screeching halt, especially when it seems like he'd rather watch the football game than talk about fertility. You're devastated every time you get your period. He shrugs and says, "We'll just try again this month. Don't worry—it will happen."

If you want to slug your husband when he says something like that, you're not the only one. Women are allowed to express their emotions more than men; we plan for things more; and we learn that being a mother is a very important part of life. Men don't get any of these messages, so they are more stoic. It can be great that at least one of you is calm, but after a while it feels like he doesn't really care, and that hurts. You wonder why he isn't more upset. Doesn't he want a baby, too? And he's wondering why you've turned into a crazy woman. Most guys fall into the "What, me worry?" camp; or, in terms of fertility, the "It will happen when it happens" camp; or, in my opinion, Camp Denial. Many guys learn early not to show vulnerability, so Camp Denial is a more friendly place than Camp Fear. Emily, 41, who'd been trying to conceive a second child for more than a year, wrote, "Don't expect your husband to 'get it' or support you—he probably won't. I admit we have a problem, but hubby does not . . . this is a problem all by itself." Amy, 32, says, "As my friends and I like to say, our husbands are always a few steps behind." This certainly isn't true all the time—some men are just as invested as their wives—but it seems to be common.

Amanda, now 40, went through several years of trying to get pregnant. "My husband was the much calmer partner as we went through infertility diagnosis and treatment," she writes. "It's fair to say that he has a more stoic approach to things that are beyond his control." They were also in different places when it came to expressing their emotions. "I liked to talk about our feelings during the process a lot more than he did, but that is kind of status quo for our marriage in all matters." And it is for a lot of us. Our guys are more willing to share their feelings than their fathers were, but they still heard that "boys don't cry." And because pregnancy doesn't happen inside them like it does for you, they feel more disconnected from the process. Although there are certainly exceptions, with most guys it's best to just realize they aren't as into it as you are, and accept that.

If you're struggling, try to schedule time to spend with your husband that gets you out of your normal routine. It could be a date, like going out to dinner or a movie, or taking a walk or bike ride together. Or you could go to a carnival, go dancing, take a shower together, go for a swim, go skiing, bring a picnic lunch to the park, or take a Sunday drive to another town. (Yes, I know these sound dorkily squeaky clean, but getting rip-roaring drunk is not the best idea when you're trying to get pregnant.) Spend time as a couple outside the house and have fun—and don't talk about fertility for once. If you have the time and the funds, getting away on vacation is even better—and it's something you'll find harder to do once you have a baby, so do it now!

Dealing with Other People (Or: Snappy Answers to Irritating Questions)

Sometimes you're holding it together just fine, or at least well enough, and then someone comes along and ruins it all for you. Hearing someone else announce their pregnancy can be very hard, even if you're happy for them. The way they tell you makes a difference, too. Sometimes people are so caught up in their own joy that they don't even think about the effect of the news on others. If pregnancy announcements make you cry or leave you tongue-tied, you can ask friends who are trying to conceive to tell you by email so that you can process the information alone or with your spouse without having to react right away. That will give you the time you need to feel happy for them.

And some people are just insensitive, even if they don't realize it. My husband and I had been trying for our first child for about four months and I was starting to wonder if there was something wrong. When a friend of mine told me that he and his wife were expecting, I was happy for them until he said, "It happened really fast. I guess we're pretty good at it." As if it were a test and they'd tried harder than we did. I had to restrain myself from snapping at him. After hearing "just relax" for the upteenth time, one IW took to asking people, "What am I supposed to do, fall asleep during sex?"

People with good intentions may ask, "When are you going to have children?" Most people who ask this are merely curious and may not fully realize how personal this question is. (It's especially unnerving when it's your mother-in-law who asks.) If you're open to talking about trying to conceive, you could say, "As soon as God sees fit to give us some," or, "Hopefully soon." But be prepared for some Nosy Nellies to then expect details. If you'd rather brush off the question, you can make a joke of it—how harsh is up to you. A few zinger answers from around the Web include:

"Well, we're waiting to see how yours turn out before we decide."

"Dang! I knew I forgot something!"

"When it's any of your business, you'll be the first to know."

"I'm holding out until I can clone myself instead."

"I already have one." (And point to your husband.)

"Just as soon as I finish smoking my last stash of weed."

Admittedly, these are better for a laugh than actual use. If it's someone you don't know well who is asking the question, it's probably better to simply change the subject. If you want to be a little more direct, you could reply with, "That's a pretty personal question. Anyway, how's your new job?" If you just can't stand it and want to teach someone a lesson, you can give *The Speech*, something like, "Thousands of couples struggle with infertility, usually in silence. I'm not going to tell you if we're one of those couples or not, because it's not your business. I'm just going to tell you how hurtful your well-intentioned question can be." I personally don't have the stomach for that kind of social humiliation, but it's true that if everyone did this, maybe fewer people would ask.

Envy . . . and Secondary Infertility

Trying to get pregnant brings out emotions you didn't know you had. One of the most common feelings is the unfairness of it all. Women—even teenage girls—who have no business raising a child get pregnant accidentally. Freaking crack addicts get pregnant! Yet when a married woman with a good job who makes responsible decisions wants a baby, the universe says, "Nah, I don't think so." It's enough to make you crazy.

It sometimes seems unfair just how easy getting pregnant was for other women. "We used the fertility monitor and when the egg came up, we did it," said one friend of mine who got pregnant on her first try even though she had irregular cycles. "I'd never charted before, but my temperature went up and never went back down," said another. I like both of these women, but I felt like they got an A+ on a test with no effort when I was stuck with a C after studying for months. For many IWs, this is the first time we've had an important goal we can't make happen by working hard. Well, we sort of can, which is why we read books, do research, buy OPKs, and chart. But after that, it's out of our hands. Especially when lots of people you know have such an easy time of it, having fertility issues makes you realize that your parents were right when they said, "Life is not fair." Damn parents. (Although now that you might be a parent soon, you might have to reconsider that statement.)

What if you already have a child—or two or three—and are having a hard time conceiving another? Women who are struggling to have even one child might not understand. Even your husband might say—like Beth's did—"We should be grateful for the child we already have." In *Inconceivable*, her memoir of secondary infertility, Julia Indichova asks, "Why does this hurt so much when I already have the most wonderful daughter in the world? How dare I lament with all those childless couples out there? Yet I can't undo the feeling of despair." Of course, you feel lucky to have the child or children you have, but it still hurts if you can't have the number you want. This is likely to be a growing problem now that women often have their first child later and the cache of having three or more children is undergoing a renaissance, especially among the upper middle class. ("Three is the new black," quipped an OB in an affluent neighborhood recently.)

Whether you are trying to get pregnant with your first child or your fourth, it's an adventure of emotions. Somewhere, in a foreign land far in the past, there were women who didn't worry about getting pregnant. They decided to "see what happens," and a baby happened—no research, a month or two of trying, no miscarriage. Some women are lucky enough to have that happen twice or even three times. For the rest of us, we have to pull out all of the weapons in our mental arsenal. Just remember that you are not in the fight alone.

CHAPTER 8

Peeing on More Sticks: The Two-Week Wait and When to Test for Pregnancy

You've successfully predicted your ovulation, done the horizontal mambo at what you think was the right time, and now . . . you wait. Waiting is no fun. Those pregnancy tests in your bathroom cabinet are calling your name—or, more accurately, your pee. Many women call this the TWW: the two-week wait.

Your best strategy for getting through the two-week wait is to distract yourself as much as possible. Tackle that tough work project, put together your photo albums, watch the movies you've wanted to see, clean the house, and stay away from the Internet, because you're just going to look at crib bedding. I mean it—take your hand off that mouse now. Pottery Barn Kids will still be there when you get back.

It's impossible to stay away from the Internet, though, and soon you'll start looking for information on how early you can test to find out if you're pregnant. Many websites—especially those in the business of selling tests—give the incorrect information that you can start testing 7, or even

6, days past ovulation (DPO). Sure, you can waste your money and emotions testing this early, but you're extremely unlikely to get a positive result. The average implantation time in the North Carolina study—detected by lab tests 100 times more sensitive than home tests—was 9 DPO. It takes two or three days after implantation for the embryo to make enough HCG (human chorionic gonadotropin, the pregnancy hormone) for even a very sensitive home pregnancy test to work. So that means the majority of women won't get a positive until 11 DPO. Only 24 percent of embryos implant before 8 DPO and thus might test positive by 10 DPO. And 13 percent of pregnancies don't even show up on the supersensitive lab tests until 11 DPO or later, so they wouldn't trip a home test until 13 DPO at the earliest. So to balance the use of expensive pregnancy tests with your own impatience, my advice is to *start testing 10 days after you ovulate or 11 if you want to be more certain*, preferably using first morning pee. I know you're thinking, "But I can't wait even a day longer. I have to know if I'm pregnant right now!" But if you test too early, you'll get a negative result even if you actually are at the very beginning of a pregnancy.

My second pregnancy illustrates why 11 DPO is not too late to start testing. The afternoon of 10 DPO, a blood HCG test came back as 8—too low for even the most sensitive pee tests. But the next morning, at 11 DPO, I got a faint positive on a pee test. (And that's how I got the news—never take a blood pregnancy test on a Friday afternoon!) And this was the *earliest* I ever got a positive. I had to wait until 13 DPO for a positive in my first and third pregnancies, after getting negatives up to that point even on sensitive tests. A FertilityFriend.com study of 93,194 charts found that the most common days to get a positive test were 13 or 14 DPO, right before when most women would expect their period.

If you don't know when you ovulated, when to test is much more of a guessing game. Some early pregnancy tests say they are accurate for more than 50 percent of pregnant women "5 days before your missed period." This translates to 10 DPO only if (1) your cycle is exactly the same length every single month and (2) your luteal phase (the time from ovulation until the start of your period) is exactly 14 days long and always is. The tests assume a 14-day luteal phase, so the day of the missed period is 15 DPO. If you ovulated late but didn't know it, 6 days before your usual period day will be too early to test. If you have a short luteal phase, it will also be too early; for an 11-day luteal phase, 6 days before the expected period is just 6 days after ovulation. (All of these calculations are enough to make you want to whine "Math class is hard!" like that horribly un-PC 1990s Barbie). This is yet another reason that it's great to chart, use OPKs, or use a fertility monitor to figure out when you ovulate: You will also know when to test, because figuring out 10 DPO is simple compared to the "days before missed period" math, especially when half of the variables are unknowns. Thus you'll avoid the ups and downs of "No, I'm not pregnant," which could a few days later turn into "Yes, I am!" Test at the right time and you'll get one correct answer.

In the range of 10 to 12 DPO there are three ways you can still get a negative even if you're actually pregnant: (1)

The embryo came fashionably late to the womb (about 40 percent of pregnancies implant at 10 DPO or later); (2) you tested later in the day, when pee is more diluted; or (3) the test wasn't sensitive enough. Remedy any or all of these (wait a day or two, test in the morning, get a more sensitive test) and you'll increase your chances of getting an accurate reading. These days, most pregnancy tests are pretty sensitive, but they usually don't publish their sensitivity in the instructions. A quick Internet search will yield a bunch of pages with lists of tests and how sensitive they are. You're looking for tests with the *lowest* HCG number, often 10 or 20 mIU/ml, which is the amount of HCG the test can detect, and you want little numbers that can find the littlest embryo.

You can get pregnancy tests many different places these days, and the more expensive ones are not usually better, just more conveniently located (like at the grocery store right next to the condoms; if they break, it's one-stop shopping). You'll find the best deals online or even at the dollar store (yes, the dollar store ones are accurate). Consider buying 5 to 10 cheap tests before you start trying. You won't jinx your chances—it's just a way to save a bunch of money. If you want a brand-name pregnancy test, your best bet is the First Response Early Result. Several scientific studies and a *Consumer Reports* study showed that it detected the smallest amount of HCG.

Another way to save money is to buy the "naked" tests that don't have a plastic cover, just a test strip. These are "dip" tests. Instead of peeing on them, you pee in a cup and then dip the test strip in. It may not be fun to contemplate your own pee, but consider it practice for when you're pregnant and will be asked to pee on demand at every doctor's visit, also into a cup. (Obstetricians love preggie pee like vampires love blood.) Some women buy little plastic pee catchers so that they will, as the website peeonastick .com puts it, "never drink from a pee cup again." The site sells its own dedicated vessel that says "My Pee Cup" on the front and quips on the back, "CAUTION: This mug is tainted with residual hormones. Drinking from it may result in obsessive line-analyzing and compulsive test-purchasing. Not to mention yellow coffee."

To relieve your anxiety, read the pregnancy test instruction booklet and make fun of it. My favorite is the illustration of the vaginaless, pubic hair–free woman putting the test between her legs while standing up—what woman pees this way? Some versions have a series of dashed lines or water droplets, presumably to represent your gorgeous pee. The instructions often say "for in vitro diagnostic use," which makes the test sound like an IVF fertility treatment. But *in vitro* just means "outside," so basically they are telling you not to stick the test up your ho-ha. It also says, "Keep out of reach of children," I guess because we don't want kids trying to copy mommy and then getting pee all over.

In all seriousness, though, read the test instructions carefully. Pregnancy tests work differently than OPK results, because the result line doesn't have to be darker than the control line. And remember that a positive pregnancy test has *two* lines, not just one. The single line, called the control line, appears to tell you that the test is working. You have to get a second line for the test to be positive.

If you test after your period is due with a sensitive test, you can use pee from any time of day as long as you didn't chug a bunch of water first. It is still possible to get a false negative after your period is due if you have a uniquely behaved embryo or didn't ovulate when you think you did. The show *I Didn't Know I Was Pregnant* is filled with stories of women who got false negative pregnancy tests, possibly because they tested too early or drank too much water, and later went on—surprise!—to deliver babies. So if you don't get your period, definitely test again to avoid being on this show—which, given its penchant for births taking place on the toilet, could have been called *I Pooped a Baby*. (That's novelist Jennifer Weiner's line, and the rest of her books are even funnier.)

Unless you used fertility drugs that include HCG, there's also no need to have a test done at your doctor's office. The pee tests at your doctor's office are the same type you can buy at the dollar store or online. A blood test isn't necessary either. It will give you the news only a day or two earlier. Blood tests detect about 5 mIU/ml of HCG, and the most sensitive pee tests go as low as 10. You might be willing to brave the needle to know a day earlier, but the time, money, and trouble involved is probably not worth it. (Okay, maybe sometimes it is. But try to resist. I know it's like putting a chocolate cake in front of a sugar addict, but try. Now excuse me while I go eat some chocolate cake. Oops, drooling.)

There is one big downside to testing early: You might be aware of an early miscarriage that otherwise would have seemed like a late period. A lot of pregnancies—the North Carolina study found about 25 percent—are lost very early, within the first four weeks after conception, and the risk is highest right after implantation. If you test early, you might find out you are pregnant only to have your period come a few days later. This is not a false positive; it's an early loss. This happened to me. I got a positive pregnancy test and excitedly showed the test to my husband and even my parents. Four days later I started to bleed, and then a test was negative later that day. I sometimes wish I hadn't known I was "almost" pregnant. I usually think more information is better, but I do wonder if I would have been better off not knowing.

Is That Really a Line or Am I Losing my Eyesight?

After "When can I test?" the most common question about testing for pregnancy is "Am I pregnant if I have to squint to see the line?" When you test early—and any time prior to 14 days after ovulation is early—even a sensitive pregnancy test will likely give you only a faint line for a positive. But if you see a colored line, even a faint one—congratulations, you're pregnant! (This is often summed up in the phrase "A line is a line.")

If you get a faint line, use a digital test next—the ones that have a little screen that says "pregnant" or "not pregnant." They are almost as sensitive as the line tests but more expensive. They are worth it for the certainty and are absolutely essential for telling husbands. Husbands do not believe faint lines. They'll say, "I don't know. I have to squint to see it. Are you sure?" This is not how you want your big announcement to go. When I got a faint line early in my first pregnancy, I knew my husband would be skeptical. So I dashed out the door, bought a digital test at the drugstore, got back, and used it before he even woke up that morning. Then I handed it to him. (His response was "What is this?"—probably what most men say when handed a pregnancy test.) Then he figured it out. After all, it said "pregnant" right on it. He was thrilled and never questioned whether I was sure I was pregnant. That night, just for fun, I showed him the other test with the faint line. He promptly said, "Are you sure that's a line?" thus confirming that the digital test was the best money I ever spent.

One warning: "Pregnant" will stay on the screen for only 24 hours, so be sure to show it to your husband before then (or take a picture) and get all of your dreamy gazing at the lovely word *pregnant* out of the way before it disappears the next morning.

What About Looking for Other Signs of Pregnancy?

Everyone loves to play the game "Am I pregnant?" based on various body signs: "Oooh, my boobs are sore; I must be pregnant." "I felt a weird twitch in my side; I must be pregnant." "My kitchen smells weird; I must be pregnant."

It's more likely that your kitchen smells weird because you need to take out the garbage. These days, home tests can detect pregnancy several days before you would feel any symptoms. On average, pregnant women experience their first symptoms 20 days after ovulation, which is more than a week after you can start testing. And many premenstrual symptoms are just like many pregnancy symptoms. Yet the Web is filled with "Am I pregnant?" quizzes. Apparently every woman has Googled "Am I pregnant?" at least once, and every site wants those money-making eyeballs. Message boards and question sites feature countless women who list their symptoms and ask, "Does this mean I'm pregnant?" These sites are somewhat entertaining, but none of this is necessary now that home pregnancy tests are accurate before your period is even due. Stop guessing and just take a pregnancy test. And if it's too early to take one, it's too early to be experiencing any symptoms.

Waiting for It

With early tests, the two-week wait is now more like the 11-day wait. But for many of us, that might as well be 11 years. Waiting sucks. It's sort of like reading an engrossing novel with a great plot, getting all wrapped up in the story, and having someone snatch it out of your hands right before the climactic scene. They then tell you that you can't read the ending for 11 days. You'd probably want to shoot them.

You're best off not shooting yourself, so you have to wait. As Carey Goldberg writes in *Three Wishes*, "This is a little like how I imagine it is to have cancer. There's all kinds of stuff going on in your body, and you're powerless to affect it, even though there's a particular outcome you desperately want to achieve. But you can't do a thing toward achieving it."

First, stop the obsessive Googling. It's not going to help.

You've done your ovulation prediction and your baby dancing, so you just have to leave it up to fate. Try to keep yourself occupied as much as possible. Organize your closet. Make a photo album. Watch lots of movies. Go to dinner. Read novels. Do everything you can to live in denial and escape thoughts of pregnancy.

If you still can't stop thinking about it, though, you're not alone. Here's how those days usually went for me:

Day 1: Temperature is up. That means I ovulated yesterday, so I can figure out how well we did this cycle. Hmmm, BD'd two days before ovulation and the day of. That's pretty good. The graph in this research article (which I have read 74 times already) says two days before has about a 30 percent chance of pregnancy. And we've been trying for four cycles, and the next graph (that I've looked at merely 53 times) says . . . crap, the average woman my age has already gotten pregnant. Damn her.

Day 2: What did those graphs say again about the chances? [Look at them 75 and 54 times, respectively].

Day 3: My temperature is not as high as I'd like. Do I have low progesterone? Maybe I should call the doctor's office now to set up an appointment.

Day 4: I wonder if any of my old charts look like this cycle. Maybe they will indicate if it's a good one. [Spend 30 minutes looking at 5 years of old charts and then 2 hours searching for similar charts on FertilityFriend.com.]

Day 5: I'm going to stop thinking about getting pregnant right fricking now. Okay, let's think about work. [15 minutes later] What was that stat on the fertility clinic website again about women my age? [Spend 30 minutes reading the webpage for the 12th time.] Damn it.

Day 6: I have *got* to stop obsessing over this. Is there any way to order more than two movies at a time on Netflix? Maybe a *Twilight* movie—that would be distracting. Except not the last one, where she has the vampire baby. Maybe *Sex in the City*. Except not the first one, where Charlotte gets pregnant after years of infertility. Maybe I'll just read a book.

Day 7: I never knew the grocery store sold five different celebrity gossip magazines. If only they didn't all have the same articles. Of course, this one doesn't even have articles, just captions under the pictures—the same pictures the other magazines have. I wonder what's on TV? Oh, look: It's another episode of *I Didn't Know I Was Pregnant*. I think *I* would know. I would have taken 2,897 tests.

Day 8: I think that graph said the chances were 30 percent, but I'm not sure. Maybe if I put a piece of paper up to the screen, I can draw a straight line and find out the exact number. Or I could print out the graph and draw the line with a ruler. That would be even better.

Day 9: First official day of toilet paper checking. And . . . there's some spotting. Is my period coming or is that implantation spotting? Google. Then look online for two hours at other women's charts that vaguely resemble mine.

Day 10: Temperature is high, but is it high enough? Should I test this morning? What if it's too early? Probably shouldn't. Oh wait—I think I should! Crap, I already peed. Have to wait until tomorrow. Unless I don't drink anything for the rest of the day. Should I do that? Is that healthy? Would that hurt the baby if I am actually pregnant?

Day 11: Might as well test. Okay, testing . . . my blood pressure is so high I hope I don't have a heart attack before I even get pregnant. That would suck.

The Longest Minute in the World

After the pee-aiming and/or the stick-dipping comes the hard part: the waiting. Again. Pregnancy tests take a minute or two to work, but it feels like hours. The dye—the blue or pink stuff that will inform you of the biggest news of your life—travels across the window like a wave in a calm pool. Meanwhile, you are anything but calm. It feels like your heart is going to beat out of your chest. Then you look at it under the brightest light possible to see if there's a second line. If it's a digital test, you stare at the hourglass symbol, trying not to blink your eyes so that you won't get the news even one millisecond later and finally see "Pregnant" or "Not Pregnant."

If it's negative, be prepared to feel, in the words of a

fellow IW, "Devastated. Pissed. Hopeless. Scared. Sad. Alone. Overwhelmed. Desperate." (Unless you are a very calm person. If so, can you please give the rest of us lessons?) If you're testing early, you can still be hopeful that tomorrow or the next day will yield a positive result. If it doesn't, you'll start thinking about the next cycle and trying again. Do your best not to get too critical of your efforts that cycle. ("If only we'd had sex every day, I'd be pregnant right now.") Yes, you'll scrutinize your chart (again), seeing if there's anything you can learn from the cycle: How many days of eggwhite did you have? How many days of "high" on the fertility monitor? How soon after the OPK or "peak" fertility did your temperature rise? You can use all of that the next time. That's the thing about trying to get pregnant: There's always a next time about 10 days away. It's a continuous roller coaster of hope and disappointment.

If the test is positive, congratulations. You've done it! You will want to hug the pregnancy test. (Don't. You'll just get pee on yourself.) I was elated the first time I got a positive pregnancy test. After feeling happy, my next thought was, "This means my tubes are open." (Clearly I had already read too much about infertility.) If you've only been trying for a few months, you will feel smug (or terrified). If you've been trying for a while, you will feel relief—you don't have to worry about getting pregnant anymore. Now you just have to worry about barfing—which, if you wanted to get pregnant, sounds pretty good, though not as good as looking at crib bedding online. Yes!

CHAPTER 9

Sad Endings: Miscarriage

"The anger I felt was like nothing I've ever experienced before. I wanted to rip my hair out and throw things across the room. I was so angry at my situation and everyone who was pregnant."

"All the dreams went down the toilet—literally. I was so sad. I cried for about 3 days. I had to put my pregnancy journal away without finishing it. I had to have an answer when my 2-year-old son asked, 'Baby in mommy's tummy?'"

"I was fortunate in how early I miscarried, but I never thought I would feel and be as emotional as I was about it. I couldn't talk about it without crying for months."

Miscarriages are surprisingly common. About 1 in 3 pregnancies don't make it to 20 weeks. (A loss after 20 weeks is considered a stillbirth.) Most of those are lost very early. About 1 out of 4 embryos that implant, and thus might show up on an early pregnancy test, don't survive past 6 weeks (4 weeks after ovulation; pregnancy weeks are traditionally counted from the woman's last period). These are often called *chemical pregnancies*—a term I hate, because it sounds like you made up being pregnant and it was just a few chemicals. *Early loss* is a better and more sensitive term. With home tests now able to detect pregnancy so early, more and more women are experiencing early losses instead of just thinking they had a late period.

After 6 to 7 weeks, when a fetal heartbeat can be seen on ultrasound, about 15 percent of pregnancies miscarry. The most common cause of both early loss and miscarriage is a chromosomally abnormal embryo, one reason the risk of miscarriage rises with age. After 6 weeks, about 10 percent of pregnancies miscarry among women under 30, about 12 percent for those 30 to 34, 18 percent for those 35 to 39, and 35 percent for those 40 to 44. The father's age is correlated with miscarriage risk, too.

Most miscarriages occur during the first trimester (the first 12 weeks), primarily before 10 weeks (because, amazingly, all of the fetal organs have already formed by then). So if something is going to go wrong, it usually goes wrong fairly early. Early pregnancy is a series of small milestones: You make it to 6 weeks; you see the heartbeat on the ultrasound at 7 weeks or so; you make it to 10 weeks; you make it to 12 weeks. If you've never had a miscarriage, you might take these steps for granted, because you don't realize that anything can go wrong. In many ways this is good, because then you're not worrying all the time. If you've miscarried before or are older and realize your increased risk, early pregnancy can be even more psychologically challenging than getting pregnant. Review the coping strategies from

Chapter 7 if you need to, and distract yourself with engrossing activities as much as possible.

How to Know If You Are Having a Miscarriage

Spotting—usually a small amount of blood, often brown—is very common during early pregnancy. So it's often difficult to know when to start worrying. If you start to see red blood that's more than just spotting, it's more likely to be a sign of miscarriage (though not always). Other signs include moderate to strong cramping, backache, or the sudden loss of pregnancy symptoms. But any of these without bleeding are usually not a problem. If you think you might be miscarrying, call your doctor, who can check to see if your cervix is open and do an ultrasound to see if the pregnancy is still viable. Most of the time, doctors can't do anything to stop a first-trimester miscarriage once it's begun. If you're further along, your doctor will tell you if anything can be done (such as putting a stitch in the cervix).

Any sign of miscarriage can be really scary, so you're likely to be superanxious if you see any spotting or bleeding. Distract yourself as much as possible and see if the spotting gets any worse. If you are very, very early in your pregnancy—within a few days of when you would have gotten your period—taking a pregnancy test again might tell you if you are losing the pregnancy. (It did for me.) Any further along, though, and a pregnancy test will still turn positive even if you're miscarrying, because the HCG levels will still be high enough.

If you weren't very far along, it's likely you will miscarry at home, getting what looks and feels like a heavy period. If you were more than six weeks along, you need to see your doctor so that he or she can make sure you miscarried completely. (If not, you may have to have a dilation and curettage—a D&C—to clear the uterus, though sometimes medication like misoprotol can be used instead.) Even if you weren't very far along, it's still an extremely good idea to get checked out by a doctor. At the very least, you can ask the many questions you're likely to have. If you miscarry at home, you should also ask your doctor if you should save the tissue for analysis. It's a gruesome question and probably not something you want to think about, much less do, but many doctors recommend it so that the cause of the miscarriage might be determined.

Let's say you continue to get spotting or bleeding and have an ultrasound to assess the pregnancy. You'll expect to get one of two answers: Yes, there is a heartbeat and everything is fine; or no, there's no heartbeat and you've miscarried. But if you get the bad news that there is no heartbeat, your doctor might want to wait a few days or even a week and repeat the ultrasound. The thinking is the due date might be off and the pregnancy might be fine. Be prepared for the sad possibility that you could end up in limbo and not get a definite answer for several more days. If you are certain of your conception date, it's likely this pregnancy will end, but it makes sense to be sure before scheduling a D&C that will end the pregnancy if you don't miscarry on your own. If you don't know when you ovulated, you might not be as far along as you think, so it pays to wait.

Many women who chart keep taking their temperature

even after they get a positive pregnancy test. Temperatures are high after ovulation and sometimes rise even higher during early pregnancy. Falling temperatures can be a sign of miscarriage. The problem is you risk freaking yourself out if you get a low temperature. You have to decide if the extra information is worth the anxiety. I got a low temperature one morning very early in my second pregnancy, 16 days after ovulation and 4 days after a positive pregnancy test, and then saw some brown spotting a few hours later. I realized that the two together were an ominous sign and prepared myself. Sure enough, I got my period by late afternoon and had to accept that the pregnancy was over. During my next pregnancy, after several days of very high temperatures, I got a lower temp. I took it again. Same result. I felt like I was going to have a nervous breakdown right then at 5:30am, huddled under the covers holding a flashlight. Somehow I made it through the day and I decided to stop taking my temperature. This time, the low temp was a false alarm and I had a healthy pregnancy with my second daughter.

Dealing with a Miscarriage

If you've followed the advice in this book, you've already cut your risk of miscarriage by eating right, not smoking, cutting down on caffeine and alcohol, and taking prenatal vitamins. And remember the surprising advice in Chapter 4: You can lower your risk of an early loss by having sex *before*, and not just *on*, the day of ovulation, because the egg is more likely to be healthy if it's fertilized right away.

But even if you've done everything right, miscarriages still happen. And if it happens to you, remember, commit to memory, and all but tattoo on your hand: It was not your fault. It's rare for a miscarriage to be caused by anything you did. And tattoo this right underneath: The chances that you will have a normal pregnancy next time are very high. Even after two losses, most women will go on to have a healthy pregnancy the next time without any intervention. My friend Sarah had a miscarriage at eight weeks, right after she told her family she was expecting. She then had an ectopic pregnancy (in which the embryo grows in the fallopian tubes, where it cannot survive). Her third pregnancy, though, was fine, and she gave birth to a healthy baby boy.

Women's reactions to miscarriages are somewhat unpredictable. Some women aren't very upset and just want to move on. But very strong feelings are common. That's an inadequate way of saying you might feel extremely angry or extremely sad. Here's another tattoo: You are allowed to feel this way. Especially if you've been trying for a long time already, the loss can be frustrating as well as sad. You probably felt such relief that your struggle to get pregnant was over—no more worrying about fertility! And then boom, you're back to the old slog of trying to get pregnant and wondering if it will ever happen.

When you miscarry, you are grieving. Just that realization alone can be helpful. You might never forget a miscarriage, but you can heal. Most studies show that grief gets better over time, with the worst of it over in six months or less. Chloe, 34, has suffered two miscarriages, which she describes as among "the most difficult experiences in my life. The only thing that made it better was time. It was and continues to be a long grieving process." When you are grieving, remind yourself that you will feel better as time goes on.

You've probably heard that grieving people go through specific stages in a certain order: denial, anger, bargaining, depression, and acceptance. Psychologists now know that it's possible to grieve in a healthy way without going through all, or even most, of those stages. For example, most people accept the reality of the situation fairly quickly and not everyone feels anger. Surprisingly, people who repress their feelings usually do just fine. You don't necessarily have to express every emotion you have about the experience. Some studies even show that people who don't dwell on their feelings do better in the long run. There is no one way to grieve.

A warning: When you're reading books or talking to doctors and nurses, you might hear the term *spontaneous abortion*. That's the technical medical term for a miscarriage; it doesn't mean that you wanted to miscarry this child. Still, this term is upsetting and I'm not sure why it's still used. Even worse, women who miscarry more than once are sometimes called *habitual aborters*. I heard a receptionist at a fertility clinic use that term when talking to a woman who'd miscarried. Not surprisingly, she looked stricken. Knowing this strange term can prepare you to hear it at an already vulnerable time.

One of the hardest things about having a miscarriage is telling people, especially because most people don't know what to say and occasionally fall back on hurtful clichés. "It's okay—you can always have another one." (But, you think, I wanted *this* baby.) "It's God's will." (Perhaps, but that seems so unfair.) "It wasn't really a person." (Not yet, but it could have been, and you might have already loved him/her.) "It's for the best—it wouldn't have been normal anyway." (That still doesn't make it fair.) "At least you already have a child." (Yes, but I wanted another one so badly.) "It's been weeks—why are you still crying?" (Would you say this to someone who lost another loved one?) As insensitive as these comments are, sometimes people say them because they don't know what else to say. They mean well. Of course, anyone who says these things and doesn't mean well is worth avoiding at all costs.

What if your husband doesn't react the way you'd like? A lot of men are stoic and want to be a rock for their wives after a miscarriage. Others just want to move forward and not think about the loss. Men aren't the ones anxiously checking the toilet paper every time they go to the bathroom or seeing the blood that means the dream of a pregnancy is over. They don't worry that they did something to cause the miscarriage. Men do feel the pain of miscarriage—it was their child, too—but they often don't feel it as acutely or in the same way as women do. Tell him you want to hear how he's feeling and let him know how sad you are. Or, if you're looking forward to moving on quickly, tell him that, too.

What Causes Miscarriages

If you have a miscarriage, you will undoubtedly wonder why it happened. Most of the time, miscarriages are abnormal embryos that just couldn't survive. It is extremely unlikely that your miscarriage was caused by having sex, picking up your toddler, worrying too much, or exercising in moderation. It's true that severe stress—such as near-starvation or a death in the family—might lead to miscarriage. But usual work stress and worrying about losing the pregnancy are unlikely to cause a miscarriage.

You will probably wonder if any treatments could help you. This is a great question for your doctor. Some doctors treat women after just one miscarriage, but others don't want to do anything until a woman has suffered two or even three. Your doctor might consider some of these treatments:

- Antibiotics (specifically erythromycin), as miscarriages are sometimes caused by infections.
- Low-dose ("baby") aspirin, especially if you have an autoimmune disorder such as lupus or thyroid disease. But ask your doctor first, as there is some concern about aspirin and birth defects.
- Blood thinners like heparin or intravenous immunoglobulin.
- Surgery to correct uterine abnormalities or remove uterine fibroids (only if you have very large or intrusive ones).
- Progesterone supplements. These have no known side effects (as long as they are natural and not synthetic progesterone), though some research has questioned whether they provide any real benefit during pregnancy. (I took them anyway with my

second child. I will never know if I actually needed them, but they helped me feel I was doing everything I could.)

Trying Again

Fortunately, you are very likely to have a successful pregnancy after one miscarriage (an 87 percent chance, which is barely different from the usual risk of miscarriage). Even if you've had two miscarriages, chances are the next pregnancy will come to term. How soon you should try to get pregnant again and how to predict your ovulation heavily depend on when you suffered the miscarriage. If you miscarried at less than six weeks, and especially five weeks, your body will most likely experience the miscarriage like a normal, though possibly heavier, period. During this next cycle right after the early loss, you can chart, use OPKs, or use a fertility monitor the same as usual. One study even showed higher chances for a successful conception in the next cycle after an early loss.

If you were further along when you miscarried but still in the first trimester, you will want to wait one cycle, though not necessarily more, to try again. Doctors used to advise waiting three or even six months, but more recently they say you can try whenever you feel ready. One study found more successful pregnancies among women who tried sooner after a miscarriage. (This was especially true among older women, where waiting six months upped the risk of another miscarriage due to age). The best solution is to wait one cycle and start trying again after you've had one normal period. Your body is still adjusting during the cycle right after the miscarriage. Many women get false positives on fertility monitors and OPKs only a week or so after their miscarriage, probably because the pregnancy hormone HCG is chemically similar to LH (the hormone that trips OPKs and gives you the "egg" on the fertility monitor). Once you've had one period after the miscarriage, though, you should be able to get normal results from these methods.

If you get pregnant again, the sad thing is that miscarriage ruins the joy of a positive pregnancy test. After our early loss, I was fortunate to get pregnant again the very next cycle. The first time, I took a digital test and was all excited to show my husband. The second time, I used a cheap line test and told my husband, "I got a positive pregnancy test this morning." He replied, "Okay." And that's exactly how I felt: Okay, let's see if this one sticks or not. As Carey Goldberg puts it in her book *Three Wishes*: "This is what miscarriage does to you; a positive pregnancy test means nothing more than a promising start. It is better than nothing, but too far from a baby for real elation."

During the first trimester of this next pregnancy, I was a complete wreck. A low morning temperature sent me into a tailspin. Every trip to the bathroom was an event featuring toilet paper checking. The day I waited for the phone call about the HCG blood test results at five weeks was one of the worst days of my life. I couldn't concentrate on anything and was on the verge of a panic attack most of the day. I finally gave up and watched a movie (*Sex and the City* . . . the first one, not the bad second one). When the office hadn't called by 4:45pm, I called them. To my immense relief, the news was good. But then I started to worry about what the ultrasound would show. In short, I took none of my own advice—and this was after being lucky enough to get pregnant naturally the cycle right after the loss. I have the deepest respect, admiration, and empathy for women who go through so much more. I didn't ever completely stop worrying during that pregnancy, and I guess that's normal.

One of the few things that helped during the first trimester of this pregnancy was talking to a friend who'd miscarried. Talking to other people didn't really help much—it's an experience that is difficult to understand if you haven't gone through it. If you don't know anyone else who has had a miscarriage, you can find a support group online. Women who have miscarried are usually very sensitive to the feelings of others who have experienced the same thing, and you will feel much less alone.

On some message boards, women call a baby conceived after a miscarriage or other loss a "rainbow baby." (Many people guess that this refers to an interracial child or the child of gay parents, but it's neither.) The term has its origins in a rainbow after a storm. And that's what a healthy baby after a loss feels like—a ray of sunshine through the clouds, eventually warming the air so much that the clouds just float away.

CHAPTER 10

When to See Your Doctor
and What to Expect When You Do

The standard advice is to try to get pregnant on your own for a year before seeing a doctor for infertility testing. My reaction to this is:

ARE YOU CRAZY? A YEAR? IT'S BEEN TWO MONTHS AND I'M LOSING MY MIND! HELP ME *RIGHT NOW*! I WANT TO BE PREGNANT SO BADLY THAT BARFING EVERY MORNING SOUNDS GOOD! CAN'T YOU SEE I'M DESPERATE HERE?

But then I am an Impatient Woman. Fortunately, the medical community is starting to come around to the idea that a year is too long to wait, particularly if a couple has been timing sex around ovulation. The guideline of a year is based on the old idea that you just throw away your birth control and fall into bed when the mood strikes. With ovulation prediction, though, the average couple under 35 is pregnant in less than three months, especially if they've had sex at the right time every cycle.

If you've been trying for more than three months, don't panic. Maybe you just haven't had your lucky cycle yet—it's a roll of the dice. It took me five cycles to get pregnant the first time even though I had charted for two years, had no known fertility issues, and was under 35. If you just can't wait—and believe me, I'm with you—you can always consider making an appointment with your OB-GYN in advance, to coincide with the month you will have been trying for six months. If your doctor's office is anything like mine, the first appointment you'll be able to get will be several months away anyway. If you get pregnant, you can always cancel—or turn it into your first pre-natal appointment.

If you've been trying to get pregnant without success, should you "stop trying" to increase your chances? This is common advice, but it's misguided. Asking a woman who wants a baby to "stop trying" is ridiculous. For one thing, it's not going to work. You've probably heard stories of couples who "stopped trying" and then finally got pregnant, but you don't hear the more common story of those who stopped and didn't get pregnant, because that doesn't make such a good story. And how exactly are you supposed to "stop try-ing" when you want to get pregnant? You'll still be thinking about it, but won't be doing anything about it. Remember that stress does not cause infertility, so "not trying" is not going to make you more fertile. And "not trying" is going to make it less likely that you have sex at the right time and thus less likely that you'll get pregnant.

If you've been trying to get pregnant for a while, you're better off trying harder: buying a fertility monitor, say, or seeing a doctor. Doing these things will also help you relieve your stress, because you'll be taking action instead of ruminating. Of course, you shouldn't "try harder" by worrying more. If you find yourself doing that, go back to Chapter 7 and try a new coping technique or two. If predicting your ovulation is your biggest source of stress, try a different method or go for the "lots of sex" plan at the beginning of Chapter 4 (or go on vacation during the middle of your cycle, to guarantee lots of sex!). But don't be surprised if not knowing when you ovulated also stresses you out. It's not "trying" that makes women anxious—it's wanting. Since you're probably not going to stop wanting a child, you have to cope as much as possible and (this is the hard part) realize that it's not fully under your control.

When Should You Seek Fertility Treatment?

Because this book focuses on natural conception, I'm not going to go too deeply into the details of fertility treatments. I'll concentrate on how to make the difficult decision of when to seek fertility treatment and what you can expect from initial visits.

Deciding when to move to fertility treatment is very difficult. Some couples try to get pregnant for years but either don't want or can't afford fertility treatment. Those are sad stories, because sometimes relatively simple medical fixes can help women get pregnant. Women who keep blogs about their fertility struggles often say they wish they'd gotten help earlier. The majority of women who seek fertility treatment don't need IVF or other high-tech procedures. Sometimes there are relatively simple solutions, such as antibiotics to clear up an infection. Other women get pregnant using IUI, which is fairly inexpensive (a few hundred dollars a try) and usually doesn't involve the extensive hormone injections that IVF does.

Other women are probably too impatient and might have gotten pregnant on their own if they'd given it six months to a year. Susan started trying to get pregnant at 37. When she wasn't pregnant after three months, she decided she had no time to lose and saw an infertility specialist. Within six months, she had IVF and got pregnant with twins. Five months after the twins' births, she was trying to figure out why her period hadn't come back, and it turned out she was pregnant. I know another woman who had triplets with IVF and then accidentally got pregnant again when the triplets were 2 years old. In both of these cases, you have to wonder if IVF was really necessary in the first place. In other cases, IVF, and nothing else, does the trick, and no one is sure why. My friend Marie started trying to get pregnant when she was 32. After fertility drugs, several failed IUIs, and surgery for fibroids, she still wasn't pregnant four and a half years later at 37. But her first try with IVF was successful, and she now has a beautiful daughter.

So when should you seek help? The general rule of thumb is to try for a year if you're 34 or younger, six months if you're 35 to 39, and three months if you're 40 or older. The irony is that older women take longer to get pregnant, yet they are told to seek treatment earlier. The idea is that they can get help "before it's too late," but entering the scary world of infertility treatment after just three months of trying when you're over 40 seems too soon, especially since one of the first things you're going to hear is just how bad your chances are because of your age.

For younger couples, though, I think a year is too long if you've been timing sex around ovulation. Doctors assume that young couples have all the time in the world and therefore often advise them to try longer on their own. This noninterventionist policy is good in some ways, but it ignores the stress around trying to get pregnant. It also ignores the time constraints some people have with their careers, finishing school, or wanting to have children spaced several years apart. So, with a year too long and three months too little, I think seeking advice after six months of well-timed sex is a nice happy medium for couples of all ages.

What to Expect When You Seek Treatment

Most of the time, the first step in fertility treatment is an appointment with your OB-GYN. This appointment may or may not be covered by health insurance; many insurance plans don't cover infertility. Some states mandate coverage for infertility, but in most there are no regulations and insurance plans vary widely. Your OB will likely run a series of blood tests for thyroid function, prolactin, and FSH (follicle-stimulating hormone—high numbers mean you might be closer to menopause). Thyroid and prolactin abnormalities can be treated with inexpensive oral medication. Little can be done about high FSH levels, but—as you might remember from Chapter 6—there's debate about how much those numbers mean for natural conception, especially if you are still having regular cycles.

Always get the exact numbers for blood test results from the nurse; don't just accept it when they say the numbers are "normal." Follow up with, "Great! Can I get the number for my records?" Then (in the words of one blogger) "run to Google." Labs have different definitions of normal, and numbers at the high or low end of the range can still indicate problems. For example, "normal" FSH could mean within the range for your age but way too high for a woman who wants to get pregnant.

For comic relief, you can amuse yourself by reading the lab slip and seeing all of the bizarre tests you could be having, such as *stone track*, *direct coombs* (does this have something to do with P. Diddy?), *occult blood*, and *rast burp*, which sounds like you ate something particularly stinky. (I'm also not sure if this is a blood test or if you have to burp on command.)

After the blood tests, the next step is usually an initial visit with a fertility specialist. It might not seem like a big deal to pay for the initial visit with a fertility doctor (about $250), but most doctors will immediately order a long list of tests such as a semen analysis, antral follicle count (see Chapter 6), more blood tests, and a hysterosalpingogram (HSG, in which a doctor injects some colored dye into your uterus to see if your fallopian tubes are open). The cost of these tests can add up quickly, often to well over $2,000.

Beyond the cost, consider how fertility testing will affect your mental health. Trying to get pregnant is so stressful that seeking help can feel like a real relief—except getting help can sometimes be even more stressful. Fertility tests are like the two-week wait, taking a pregnancy test, and waiting for an important call all wrapped into one. There's the stress of taking the test itself, the worry of waiting for the results, and the effort to hold it together once you get the results. If they're not normal, you might have the sad, almost shameful feeling that you are broken or flawed, and you will face the prospect of treatment with uncertain results. If they're all normal, it's frustrating because then you don't know what's wrong and how to fix it. If you want a quick halfway solution to all of the tests, have your husband get a semen analysis if you haven't already (for more on semen analysis, see Chapter 1). It is nonintrusive and inexpensive and can diagnose 40 percent of fertility problems. It's best to get one from a doctor rather than using a home test, as the home tests are incomplete (often measuring volume but not motility).

The longer you've been trying, the more it's worth it to do the tests. You might finally solve the mystery of why you're not getting pregnant and be able to settle on a treatment plan with your doctor. If your tubes are blocked, for example, IVF is your best option. If you're not ovulating or have very long cycles, you can try Clomid, an inexpensive medication that helps women ovulate. If your husband's semen analysis showed issues, varicocele surgery or an IUI might work. Men can also try supplements like ProXeed. Among men with low sperm counts, 21 percent of their partners got pregnant naturally after three months of taking ProXeed, compared to only 2 percent without.

Many fertility treatments have downsides. Clomid, though inexpensive and easy to take, can dry up cervical mucus. (You can take Mucinex or use PreSeed lubricant if that happens.) There's also about a 10 percent chance of twins with Clomid, and you can only take it for six months. IUIs have a success rate of only 15 percent per cycle, even lower if you're over 35. And IVF, though it boasts success rates near 50 percent a cycle for women under 35, is very expensive ($10,000 or more a cycle) and involves lots of unpleasant stuff like giving yourself hormone injections. If you're over 35 or especially 40, the success rate of IVF is considerably lower. For most women over 40, natural conception might be more likely to lead to pregnancy than IVF. I am not saying that fertility treatments are bad—for many, many couples they are the best and sometimes only route to pregnancy—but couples should know all of the risks and benefits.

When you are thinking about getting fertility treatment, you have to strike a delicate balance between your impatience and entering a medical system that can be inherently stressful. As soon as you see a fertility specialist, trying to get pregnant becomes an unpleasant medical procedure instead of sex in the bedroom. You're pulled into the anxious world of a fertility clinic, where you're likely to enter the standard program of Clomid for three cycles, IUI for three cycles, and then on to IVF. As Dr. Alice Domar's research shows, fertility treatment in itself can lead women to become depressed, which further hampers their fertility. (Remember that it's depression, not anxiety, that is linked to fertility problems.) And as Dr. Sami David relates in his book *Making Babies*, many doctors don't search for the causes of infertility thoroughly enough, and many couples get the frustrating diagnosis of "unexplained" infertility.

No one knows what is wrong, so the doctors assume IVF will fix it. Dr. David relates several stories of long-infertile couples with infections, high mercury levels, and lifestyle issues who got pregnant naturally within a few months once the problem was found and remedied. So for some couples, the trick is in finding the right doctor who will look at all the possible causes of infertility.

What if no obvious cause can be found or no cause other than your age? See another doctor to get a second opinion; perhaps he or she will find the cause. If your infertility is still unexplained, consider trying on your own for longer. One study found that half of couples who didn't get pregnant during their first year of trying succeeded during the second year without medical intervention. Fertility treatments are a slippery slope, starting gradually with tests and building until you're giving yourself injections and paying tens of thousands for IVF. As Peggy Orenstein writes in her fertility memoir *Waiting for Daisy*, "The potential, however slim, that the next round might get you pregnant creates an imperative that may not have otherwise existed. If you didn't try it, you'd always have to wonder whether it would have worked. That's how you lose sight of your real choices, because the ones you're offered make you feel as if you have none."

Who Should You See for Infertility Treatment?

Most women who are having trouble getting pregnant go first to their OB/GYN. That works very well for the initial blood tests. Once you proceed to actual fertility treatment, you may have the choice of continuing with your OB or seeing a doctor who specializes in infertility (often called reproductive endocrinologists, or REs). Some OBs will prescribe Clomid for a few cycles and hope that does the trick. If you can afford it, it's often better to see an RE. They are set up to run all of the necessary tests, so you won't end up taking Clomid when your tubes are blocked and what you really need is IVF. And most REs monitor women taking Clomid using ultrasound to make sure they aren't making too many eggs (called ovarian hyperstimulation), whereas most OBs don't. However, some OBs can take you all the way through to IUI, so if you like your OB it might be worth sticking with him or her. (As one friend of mine put it, "I got knocked up by my OB.")

If you decide to see an RE, don't automatically go to the one your OB recommends. Most REs operate outside of insurance-based medical groups, and one of the few upsides to paying out of pocket is you can choose any doctor you want. Ask friends for referrals, check online sites like Angie's List or message boards, and so on. You can also learn a lot about a practice by reading its website—not just the positive advertising but what it chooses to focus on. Good signs include a focus on patient education and highlights of research going on at the clinic. Most sites include pictures of babies born from treatment, but take a look at the pictures and presentation: Are these just pictures, or do they look like slick advertising? If you expect you'll be moving on to IVF, you can check the clinic's IVF success rates online (though keep in mind that some clinics specialize in older women or tougher cases, which can bring down their stats).

Technical prowess is not the only consideration in choosing an RE. Some fertility clinics can seem like assembly lines, with the REs treating each patient in the same predictable procession from Clomid to IUI to IVF, sometimes without finding the underlying problem. In *Inconceivable*, Julia Indichova writes about seeing a doctor who clearly didn't remember who she was from one visit to the next. Ellie, 37, saw an RE who promised to answer all of her questions at the end of the appointment. The RE gave a boilerplate speech about fertility, did an ultrasound, wrote the orders for the usual tests, and then left without answering any of Ellie questions. Some clinics also give off a vibe of looking out for the bottom line a little too much. Heather, 39, saw several REs and settled on a doctor who, as she put it, "we felt was helping us and not just taking our money."

Other clinics, however, have doctors who are truly dedicated to personalizing a treatment plan, and those are worth seeking out if you can find them through referrals. Because infertility is so stressful, finding an RE who is pleasant and sensitive to the emotional side of infertility is key. My friend Jackie loved her doctor because he listened to what she and her husband wanted, but still made his own recommendations based on his experience. My friend Helene's RE liked to wear his cowboy hat for good luck when he did IVF transfers, which also made for good jokes given she was using OB stirrups herself at the time (her own cute little cowgirl was born nine months later).

If you can find an RE who helps you feel comfortable,

it will make a big difference to you psychologically. As with any medical specialty, there are doctors with great bedside manners and those who seem to have no clue how grating they are. "Most of the fertility doctors I saw seemed like they'd had *in*sensitivity training," my friend Marie told me soon after the doctor doing her IUI said, "There's no way this is going to work" as he was inserting the catheter. Doctors sometimes speak dispassionately and even coldly about fertility problems, seemingly oblivious to just how emotional these issues are for the couples involved. They've been trained to do procedures and sometimes seem to forget that these are actual people, or they have so many patients with so many problems that they don't have enough empathy to go around.

If you seek fertility treatment, do everything you can to nurture yourself mentally and physically. Keep using your favorite coping strategies and try new ones. Joining a support group for infertile couples such as Resolve is an excellent idea, especially if you can meet other women in person and feel like you are not alone. You might not have voluntarily joined the sisterhood of women struggling with infertility, but you will find that their embrace is close and warm.

CHAPTER 11

Congratulations, and Get Ready to Go to Bed at 8pm: After You're Pregnant

So your digital pregnancy test says "Pregnant"—congratulations! You are now officially allowed to look at nursery furniture online, dream up names for your future child, and be happy that you don't have to worry about getting pregnant anymore (now you get to worry about labor).

Enjoy the next few weeks. At this stage your pregnancy is probably a secret between you and your husband. And you'll get a break of a week or two between the positive test and getting the yucky symptoms of the first trimester. I started getting really tired at about five and a half weeks into my first pregnancy, which happened to be the day before we moved. I'm surprised I was able to get off the couch long enough for the movers to load it into the truck, and I got right back on it as soon as they set it down in the new house. About a week after that, I couldn't figure out why the new fridge smelled so bad. Then I realized that morning sickness had struck.

Of course, some women feel fine during their first trimester. I even know one woman who didn't realize she was pregnant until she was four months along. I hate these women. Okay, not really hate, more like I am so intensely envious it feels like hate. But most women don't feel well their first trimester in one way or another. It's just something you have to go through to reach your goal of having a healthy baby. You get a reprieve of sorts in your second trimester, when the nausea and tiredness have mostly passed but you're not too big yet. Then in the third trimester, not being able to pick things up off the floor gets old really quickly, and you just want it to be over.

But you'll also feel very happy you're finally pregnant—and rightly so. Before I had children, I heard parents complain so much it was downright frightening. It was almost like they were having a contest to see how bad they could make parenthood sound: You don't get any sleep until they're 12; you have no time to yourself anymore; sex will be a distant memory; and (my favorite) your life will never be the same again. Then, as a finale, they would say, "But it's all worth it."

Sure, I thought, you say that because you can't exactly take your kid back to the store. Parenthood is pretty irrevocable, so you might as well see the bright side even if there isn't one. After I had kids, I learned two important things. First, a lot of the complaints were exaggerations. Yes, having kids is a lot of work and there are downsides, but there are ways to manage them. Second, to my surprise, it really was worth it. I realized that parents have a hard time talking about the upsides of having children because those positives are so hard to put into words, and when you do you sound like a cheesy greeting card commercial. Even when my first daughter was nursing every three hours around the clock, the joy I felt when I held her made up for all those intrusions into my sleep time. And within a few months, she was sleeping through the night. A few months after that, she was in daycare and I could once again have lunch without eating with one hand and holding her in the other. The discomforts were temporary; the joy only grew.

This is sometimes tough to remember when you're pregnant. That's true with your first, when it's all new and scary and you haven't yet experienced loving your own child. It's also true with your second, because pregnancy symptoms are sometimes worse the second time around, and you have already learned how to worry like a mother. Being pregnant, as opposed to trying to get pregnant, requires a lot less action. Growing a person takes a lot of energy, but it's mostly involuntary energy, kind of like breathing. Yes, you have to continue to eat right, get your exercise, and see your doctor, but a lot of pregnancy is waiting. You wait to feel better. You wait to find out if you're having a boy or a girl. You wait to find out how the birth goes.

One thing you can do is read about labor. There are many choices in labor and birth, and you will be better prepared if you gather as much information as you can. Your doctor can tell you a lot—especially about the hospital procedures—but doctor appointments are fairly short even during pregnancy. If you want to go natural, you'll definitely want to take classes and read a lot about the experience, and you might want to hire a labor coach (usually called a *doula* . . . no, it doesn't rhyme with koala; it's pronounced doo-la). If, however, you're terrified about the pain of labor, just plan on getting an epidural as soon as possible. You'll still want to learn the natural childbirth techniques of deep breathing and so on—you'll need them for the car ride and when you first get to the hospital—but there's no real reason to fear childbirth pain in this era of epidurals on demand. (Though I am still waiting for a minivan model that comes with an anesthesiologist as an optional feature—I could have used that during my too-quick second labor.) But don't spend so much time reading about birth that you neglect reading and learning about babies and children. Birth lasts at most a day, but parenting lasts for the rest of your life!

One small piece of advice about birth that you might not expect to hear from me: *Don't* be impatient about it. When you've followed the advice in this book and precisely planned your child's conception with meticulous type A detail, it might seem logical to apply the same organized approach to labor and delivery. It can be tempting to schedule an induction when you're sick of being pregnant or request a C-section because you're scared of labor. But birth is usually healthiest for mother and baby when it is *not* planned. Inductions don't always work (which usually means a C-section), and a C-section, planned or not, is major abdominal surgery.

I had a C-section with my first daughter because she wouldn't come out after many hours of pushing. (I told her about this, and she now announces with kindergartener authority, "I got *stuck*!") With my second daughter, though, I had a quick labor and a vaginal birth. I can't even describe how much better the vaginal birth and recovery was compared to the C-section. I was walking normally within hours; after the C-section, I shuffled for days and had to move very slowly when doing the simplest things like getting into bed or going to the bathroom. I couldn't give my first daughter a bath for months because I couldn't kneel on the floor. Of course, I am grateful that a C-section was available to rescue me and my daughter when all other options had been exhausted. But, having had both types of births, I would never choose a C-section if a vaginal birth were an option. I could have had another C-section the second time, scheduled it for a convenient day and time, and gotten over my impatience with being pregnant and huge. But when patience means you don't have surgery, there's something to be said for it.

You are probably finishing this book before you get pregnant, wondering what the future will bring. Now you know: You're not the only one stressing out about getting pregnant. But you also have the best information for making that happen.

Have you ever tried the endlessly entertaining game of adding "in bed" to the end of the statement in your Chinese fortune cookie? Yours reads something like this: "Your future will involve much peeing on sticks and lots of fun" . . . in bed. Before you know it, you'll be feeding a baby in that bed, sleep deprived but grateful for every minute with the little miracle in your arms.

The Really Impatient Woman's Guide to Getting Pregnant:

Most of the Advice, All of the Truth,

with a Few of the Jokes

- Take prenatal vitamins one to two months before you start trying.
- Follow the SOS diet for fertility: spinach, olives, and salmon. Spinach stands for fruits, vegetables, and whole grains. Olives stand for a Mediterranean diet: lots of vegetables, a little olive oil, and fish. Salmon means low-mercury, high omega-3 fish.
- Track your ovulation by charting, OPKs, a fertility monitor, or all three.
- A woman under 35 who knows her fertile time and has sex then will get pregnant about 65 percent of the time, not the 25 percent often mentioned online and in books.
- Have sex one or two days before ovulation. (The day of ovulation is less fertile and more likely to lead to an early loss.)
- To have a boy, have sex two or more days before ovulation. To have a girl, have sex the day of ovulation. Yes, this

is the opposite of Shettles' method. The difference: He never did a systematic study and other researchers did.

- The commonly mentioned statistic that only 65 percent of women 35 to 39 will be pregnant within a year comes from birth records from 17th-century France. (Really.) More recent studies find that over 85 percent of 35- to 39-year-old women are pregnant after a year of regular sex.
- Being worried, stressed out, and anxious will *not* make you infertile. (So, "Just relax and you'll get pregnant" is *not* true.) But feeling stressed is still no fun. Cope by learning how to stop rumination, combating depression naturally, and challenging negative thoughts.
- Seduce your husband with lingerie and words, not by waving your OPK. Anything you just peed on is not romantic.
- The best day to *start* testing for pregnancy is 10 days after ovulation. Earlier than that and you're very likely to get a false negative. But don't stop testing that day, because you might not get a positive, even with a very sensitive test, until 13 days after ovulation or even later.
- You can control a lot of trying to get pregnant, but you can't control the end result of getting pregnant. Learn as much as you can, but then try to distract yourself and concentrate on having a good time.

Abbreviations Decoded

How to Acronym with the Rest

of the Crowd

AF = Aunt Flo = your period

BBT = basal body temperature (your temp right when you wake up)

BD = baby dancing (otherwise known as sex)

BFN = big fat negative

BFP = big fat positive (or big fricking positive)—usually on a pregnancy test

BMI = body mass index

CD = cycle day

CM = cervical mucus

DH = dear husband (Some guess it stands for damn husband. Could also stand for designated hitter.)

DHEA = dehydroepiandrosterone

DPO = days past ovulation

DS or DD = dear son or dear daughter

EDD = estimated date of delivery

EWCM = eggwhite cervical mucus (the fertile stuff)

FSH = follicle-stimulating hormone

HCG = human chorionic gonadotropin (what a pregnancy test detects; can also be a shot used in fertility treatment)

HSG = hysterosalpingogram (to see if your fallopian tubes are
    open)
HPT = home pregnancy test
IUD = intrauterine device
IUI = intrauterine insemination
IVF = in vitro fertilization
IW = Impatient Woman
LH = lutenizing hormone (detected by OPKs and fertility
    monitors)
LOL = laughing out loud
LP = luteal phase (the time between ovulation and your period)
MC or m/c = miscarriage
MIL or FIL = mother-in-law or father-in-law
O = ovulation (not orgasm, sadly)
OB = obstetrician
OPK = ovulation predictor kit
PCOS = polycystic ovarian syndrome
pg = pregnant
POAS = pee on a stick
RE = reproductive endocrinologist (a doctor specializing in
    fertility issues)
TTC = trying to conceive
TWW or 2WW = two-week wait, the time between ovulation
    and your period when you are waiting to find out if you are
    pregnant

Countdown to Trying

Nine months to one year in advance

- ✎ Look into your workplace's maternity leave policy, and plan when to get pregnant around it if necessary.
- ✎ Find out what coverage your health insurance offers for pregnancy, birth, and well-baby visits. Change your health plan if necessary.
- ✎ Discontinue birth-control shots (e.g., DepoProvera).
- ✎ If you're overweight, start a diet and exercise program to get to a healthier weight before you start trying.
- ✎ If you're underweight and have short or irregular cycles, gain weight until your cycles normalize (often at a BMI of 20).

Six months in advance

- ✎ Discontinue birth-control pills (if your natural cycles are irregular, or you have been on the pill for longer than two years).
- ✎ Make an appointment to see your doctor for a "preconception" visit (get tested for infections, check your immunity to rubella, and ask your doctor about how any conditions you have or prescription drugs you take would impact getting pregnant or staying pregnant).
- ✎ Start charting to learn about your cycles.

- Start a program to quit smoking.
- Stop using recreational drugs (for example, marijuana stays in your system for several months, so quit now).

Three months in advance

- Discontinue birth-control pills if you haven't already.
- Start charting your cycles if you haven't already.
- Start eating a healthier diet (you are what you ate three months ago, so it's not too early).
- Update your immunizations (especially DPT—diphtheria, pertussis, and tetanus).
- Talk your husband into making an appointment for a semen analysis.
- Remind hubby not to sit in hot tubs over 99 degrees.
- Have hubby start a men's multivitamin (zinc and vitamin C are the most important).

Two months in advance

- Start taking prenatal vitamins and supplements.
- Start reducing (or eliminating) alcohol use (that means hubby, too).
- Start reducing caffeine use.
- Stop taking any prescription drugs that aren't safe when you're trying to conceive and substitute safer alternatives if available.
- If you engage in a very high level of exercise (especially running), start tapering down your miles or hours.

One month in advance

- Buy a fertility monitor and test sticks or OPK sticks.
- Buy several pregnancy tests.

↦ See your dentist and get your teeth cleaned and any other work done (you will *not* want to do this during the first trimester!).

The cycle you start trying

↦ Eat healthy food as much as possible.
↦ Eliminate or reduce alcohol and caffeine.
↦ Consult your calendar to determine your most likely fertile days.
↦ Review Chapter 4 to see the best times to have sex.
↦ Have fun!

The Impatient Woman's Shopping List

Fortunately, trying to get pregnant naturally is usually not as expensive as an actual baby—you can get a fertility monitor, the most expensive item on this list, for the price of an average car seat, and less if you buy it used. Even so, you don't need everything on this list—it will depend on your own budget and your chosen ovulation prediction method. But feel free to bring this list to the store as your own personal preconception registry.

1. Prenatal vitamins with at least 800 micrograms folic acid and 10 milligrams vitamin B6. My favorite: Rainbow Light's Complete Prenatal System. It's the only prenatal vitamin I've found with enough calcium, so you'll save on buying calcium supplements. Ginger juice and probiotics also seemed to help with morning sickness.
2. Omega-3 fish oil supplements. My favorite: Costco's Kirkland brand, 1,000 milligrams, once a day.
3. CoQ-10 supplements. These range from 30 to 100 milligrams. Trader Joe's has a good one.
4. Any other supplements you want to try, such as DHEA.
5. A digital thermometer with a readout to two decimal places.
6. A Clearblue Easy fertility monitor and a three-month supply of test sticks.

7. Ovulation predictor strips. Start with 15. Buy them online, where they are often cheaper; get the plain strips and a plastic pee cup (instead of the plastic-encased strips) to save money. A good source: early-pregnancy-tests.com.

8. Regular ("line") pregnancy tests. Start with 10, and again buy plain strips.

9. Digital pregnancy tests. Buy a two-pack. Use one after you get a positive on a line test, to tell your husband. The second one is a nice backup and good to take a few days after the first one for reassurance.

10. Preseed lubricant, if you usually use lubricant.

11. The books from Appendix H (Further Reading) that interest you.

12. Your favorite aphrodisiac, whether that's lingerie, candles, or a vacation.

13. A steel or non-BPA plastic water bottle, and glass bowls for cooking in the microwave.

14. A rice cooker and a vegetable steamer for making healthy food.

Food Ideas

I purposely didn't call this appendix "recipes," unless you consider "take cereal box out of pantry; pour milk" and "remove pizza from freezer, take out of box, and put in oven" recipes. Instead, these are just a few healthy food ideas that require minimal effort and time (I am an Impatient Cook as well as an Impatient Woman).

1. **Healthy yogurt:** Buy plain low-fat or nonfat yogurt and mix with half a container of baby food (my favorite: Gerber's Berry Banana, though other fruits work, too). You'll avoid the massive amounts of artificial sugar in most yogurt and sweeten your yogurt with pureed fruit.
2. **Easy veggies:** Buy a vegetable steamer (I think the free-standing ones are easiest). Follow the directions, and it will cook veggies in the healthiest way possible. Buy pre-chopped veggies in a bag at the grocery store and there's virtually no effort involved. Works especially well for broccoli, cauliflower, pea pods, and green beans.
3. **Easy rice:** Same goes for rice—buy a rice cooker to do the work for you. Buy bulk brown rice, wild rice, barley, quinoa, or rice medleys—look for 3 grams or more fiber per serving—add water according to the rice cooker's directions, do something else for about 30 minutes, and serve perfectly cooked rice. Just don't lose the special measuring cup like I did.

4. **Sweet potatoes galore:** A lot of stores sell sweet potato spears in a bag. These can be grilled (yay—hubby does the work!) or baked. I've put them in a glass baking pan with some olive oil and a little salt and pepper and baked them. They're softer this way than when grilled but taste even better. You can also buy frozen sweet potato fries—use them as a healthier substitute for regular fries (sweet potatoes have lots of vitamin A and other health benefits).

5. **Easy bok choy:** Chop the lower, white part off baby bok choy, leaving just the leaves. Put a little olive oil, salt, and garlic powder in a skillet and cook box choy on medium to high heat until it's about one-third brown and crispy (with the rest cooked down but still green). Extremely healthy and at least approaches tasty.

6. **Grilled fish:** Almost all fish tastes great just grilled on an indoor (say, Foreman) or outdoor grill. Add a little lemon pepper for flavor, or mango or other salsa for drier fish like mahi mahi or halibut. For salmon, pour soy sauce on it and let it sit for about 15 minutes before you grill it. Trader Joe's Soyaki sauce is especially good on salmon.

7. **Grilled or baked chicken:** Here's two ideas. Chicken works well on an indoor or outdoor grill—add some chicken seasoning if you like. Try packaged chicken breasts first, and if you're not a fan try thighs—they aren't as dry. My favorite for baked chicken is old-school: Shake and Bake. The package has everything you need outside of the actual chicken breasts, and shaking the bag is oddly fun. The breading adds only a minimal amount of fat and locks in moisture, which makes the chicken taste better. Yet another one that takes only a few minutes to prepare.

8. **Turkey is your friend:** If you have a favorite dish made with ground beef (say, tacos), substitute ground turkey. It tastes almost the same, and it's leaner and better for you. Even more so: turkey burgers have considerably less fat

and more protein than beef burgers. Put it on a whole-wheat bun and you're all set.

9. **Spinach instead of iceberg lettuce:** If you eat sandwiches (at home or at a place like Subway), put raw spinach on them instead of lettuce. You'll get a lot more nutrients and fiber. Iceberg lettuce is a virtual nutrition desert, but spinach is the rain forest. Darker lettuce is better than iceberg, but spinach is another notch up in benefits. If you're making your sandwiches at home and are pressed for time, buy the bagged salads of spinach. If the thought of spinach makes you think of gross-looking, Popeye-strained stuff, don't worry—raw spinach tastes and looks much better, and on a sandwich you barely taste it.

10. **Add your veggies:** If you buy a prepared frozen pasta dish, make it a little healthier by adding some frozen broccoli (or other veggie) before you cook it. It will still be just as easy and fast to make, but you will get more veggies.

Troubleshooting

Not all of us have perfect cycles, youth on our side, or an easy time getting pregnant. The table below gives some solutions to common problems you might encounter.

Problem or Issue	Solutions
Difficulty seeing ovulation on your chart	1. Make sure you have a sensitive thermometer and that you're taking your temperature at about the same time each morning. 2. Use a fertility monitor or OPKs to see if you're making LH, which usually triggers ovulation. 3. If you have very long cycles and think you might not be ovulating, see your doctor, who will likely prescribe Clomid.
Ovulation, but consistently long cycles	1. Follow the diet recommendations in Chapter 2 for a few months to see if this improves your cycles. 2. Try for 3 cycles or so first, charting and using a fertility monitor to time sex. 3. If that doesn't work, see your doctor and ask if Clomid might work for you or if you need to be tested for PCOS.

Problem or Issue	Solutions
Short luteal phase (10 days or less)	1. Don't freak out—having a short luteal phase might not make any difference in getting pregnant quickly. Try for 3 to 6 months before you do *anything*, including at-home supplements, which could make things worse. 2. If you've had 6 months of ovulation-focused sex, see your doctor to try to get a prescription for supplemental progesterone. 3. Or get the usual fertility tests to rule out other issues first.
Being over 35 years old	1. Unless you're over 42, odds are on your side that you'll be able to get pregnant on your own within 6 months to a year. Consider doing some fertility tests, particularly the semen analysis, before you start trying. 2. Get a fertility monitor to perfect your timing and make the most of your chances. 3. See your doctor for tests if 6 months of ovulation-focused sex haven't done the trick.
Lack of eggwhite cervical mucus	1. Realize this may be due to coming off the pill or breastfeeding. 2. Check internally instead of externally (after washing your hands, of course). 3. If it's still AWOL, try PreSeed or Mucinex. 4. If none of this works after 6 months, see your doctor.

Problem or Issue	Solutions
Abnormal semen analysis results	1. Your husband's doctor should be able to advise him about the next steps. Make sure they involve getting tested for infections, as those are usually easy to fix. 2. If there's no way to fix the problem, ask if IUI might work. If the answer is no, IVF with sperm injection gets around almost all sperm issues.
Blocked fallopian tubes	IVF is usually the suggested solution for this problem.
Uterine fibroids	Fibroids usually don't prevent women from getting pregnant. If you know you have fibroids and have tried for 6 months or more, see your doctor.
Hypothyroidism	As long as you're taking your thyroid medication consistently, hypothyroidism probably won't cause problems in getting pregnant. Ask your doctor if you should take baby aspirin in your first trimester; some doctors recommend it if you have thyroid antibodies.

More Details on Having a Girl or a Boy: How Shettles Got It Wrong

Before we tried to get pregnant with our first child, I read about the Shettles method (to have sex far from ovulation for a girl, close for a boy) and then about studies showing there was no relationship between sex timing and having a girl versus a boy. In conceiving all three of my children, I was more concerned with just getting pregnant. So we didn't try to influence the sex of our children through timing, and I didn't think about the issue much again until I started doing the research for this book. I had no opinion going into this debate—just an interest in trying to ferret out the truth.

My original plan was for *The Impatient Woman's Guide* to have only a very short section on choosing the sex of your baby, possibly containing just one word: MicroSort (the sperm-sorting technique with proven effectiveness). But I decided I should read as many studies on the topic as possible. The more I read, the more it seemed that Shettles' theory was not just wrong, but that the opposite timing (far away from ovulation for a boy, close for a girl) actually worked better. Thus, using the Shettles method might actually be more likely to result in a child the *opposite* sex from what you wanted. Dr. Shettles' book has sold an incredible 1.5 million copies, so that's big news.

I've summarized the studies supporting the opposite timing in Chapter 5. I also read the updated 2006 version of Landrum Shettles and David Rorvick's book *Choosing the Sex of Your Baby:*

The Method Best Supported by Scientific Evidence. I thought it was important to consider what Shettles and Rorvick had to say, both about Shettles' own evidence and about the evidence suggesting his method was wrong. (Dr. Shettles died in 2003, but the book was also updated in 1996.) That's the focus of this appendix.

Shettles' Evidence

The biggest problem with Shettles' theory is he had no scientific evidence of his own—he never published data on his sex selection technique in a scientific journal article, the basic requirement for research to be part of the scientific body of knowledge. Journal articles are read by other scientists and an editor (in a process called "peer review"). These experts make sure the studies are done correctly, with unbiased samples and proper methods. Publishing results in a book isn't the same, as it hasn't been peer reviewed by other scientists and thus isn't held to the high scientific standards of a journal article. Shettles' one article on sex selection presented his theory, but no actual data on whether you're more likely to get a boy or a girl when you have sex at different times relative to ovulation. The book claims a 75 to 80 percent success rate for his method based on questionnaires from readers, admitting that they don't have the "large office staff" or "sizable funding" necessary to follow up with the readers who submitted an initial questionnaire saying they wanted to try for a boy or a girl (p. 43). That means Shettles had to rely on readers voluntarily sending in their questionnaires *after* the births of their children. Because the happy customers were probably more likely to write back—and the unhappy customers possibly unwilling to even admit to their unhappiness—this could substantially bias the results. When the results determine whether your data are in the sample at all, the data become virtually meaningless. This large flaw may be why Shettles never published his results in a medical journal.

Shettles offered lots of indirect evidence for his method,

like deep-sea divers being more likely to have girls (supposedly because the girl sperm are hardier) and results from artificial insemination, which of course is a very different setup from natural conception. Shettles acknowledged that this evidence is only indirect (p. 84), which it is—none of this really matters for couples trying to time sex.

Shettles discussed some of the medical journal articles finding that the opposite timing works better, and dismissed them. In some cases he made valid points about the shortcomings of the other studies, but these shortcomings are not as large as those in Shettles' own reader surveys. Shettles did not even mention some of the studies most damaging to his theory, such as the Australian study showing that couples who tried his method were more likely to get babies of the *opposite* sex.

As for the other studies:

᠅ The Shettles book claims that the New Zealand study by John France "used retrospective methods to try to determine the day of ovulation" (p. 98). In fact, the New Zealand study used three methods to determine ovulation (mucus, temperature, and LH in urine), and none of those measures were retrospective (meaning collected later and relying on memory; in fact, they were all collected in real time. It's hard to imagine how a urine test could ever be retrospective—you're recalling your pee?)

᠅ Shettles wrote that Guerrero's data on natural conception were based on women trying to avoid pregnancy, but Guerrero's paper notes his sample included both women trying to get pregnant and those charting to avoid pregnancy. Shettles then criticizes Guerrero's use of the women's charts, but of course charting is likely the most common way that women use Shettles' own method (as Shettles and Rorvik note themselves in pp. 123–139 of their book).

᠅ Shettles claimed that Zarutskie's meta-analysis concluded that "all six studies . . . contain no information that can be useful for sex selection by average couples" (p. 98). In actuality, Zarutskie's paper concluded that sex timing for sex selection—the crux of Shettles' method as well—is not practical because the differences were so small (similar to the 45 percent vs. 55 percent results I found in my own meta-analysis of all of the studies). Saying the difference is small is not the same as saying that the studies have no useful information. Here is Zarutskie's exact language: "The timing of intercourse in relation to ovulation and subsequent fertilization appears to influence the sex ratio. More females are conceived when coitus occurs relatively close to ovulation, and more males are conceived when the sperm or egg is in the reproductive tract for a relatively longer time before conception. The influence of coital timing on the sex ratio is overall quite subtle and is not a practical method to alter the sex ratio for individual couples" (p. 903). Zarutskie did not say the studies are not useful or valid, but that they show small differences.

Shettles and Rorvik do mention four studies published in medical journals that support the Shettles method. However, all four had some problem that prevented them from being included in the meta-analyses (either the two journal article meta-analyses or the one I did for this book). The first paper, published in 1972, is only available in Polish. The second paper is in French. The Polish paper (according to a report in a nonjournal, the *Medical World News*, which Shettles quoted) involved 322 couples, and the French paper—for which an English one-paragraph summary is available in the database Medline—included 100 (though the abstract wasn't clear about how many actually got pregnant). Without enough details on the studies and their methods, it's hard to say whether they could be included in the meta-analyses if they were translated. Neither of the meta-analyses published in medical journals chose to include them. With most other studies finding the opposite timing working, including these foreign studies would only push the results closer to an even 50/50 split.

So if we include these two studies along with all of the others to be as fair and inclusive as possible, we're back to the conclusion that sex timing doesn't make any difference for the gender of the baby.

The third paper Shettles and Rorvik mention is available in English; it found that of the 31 women in the study, conducted in Singapore, all wanted boys but only 14 had them. It notes that only 6 women used the method correctly, of which 66 percent had boys. Yet 4 out of 6 could easily have been due to chance, and entering these results into the meta-analysis did not change the results because it's such a small number. The paper concludes that the researchers' sex selection clinic was a failure. The last article reports on 10 births, all of which were of the preferred sex. However, the article does not specify how the day of ovulation was identified, and the instructions given to the couples were wildly incorrect—for example, saying that cervical mucus is the most fertile one to two days *after* ovulation (it's one or two days *before*). It also suggests that couples wanting a boy postpone sex until after ovulation, which is very unlikely to result in pregnancy at all. My favorite sentence from the article: "It should be impressed on both parties that the procedure is a scientific exercise and not an emotional or erotic skirmish." Try *that* line on your husband the next time you want to have baby sex.

So, overall, I don't think that Shettles presented any information in his book that refutes the studies finding that the opposite timing works better, nor did he present any good hard data showing that his method actually works. As I noted in Chapter 5, you're better off trying the opposite timing, and maybe doing a few of the dietary changes. It's not guaranteed to work, but at least you'll tip the odds in your favor—based on the best evidence available.

Further Reading

Here's my Impatient Woman list of books, with what's good and occasionally not so good about each. I've included only the best here—those that have more information than I could quickly summarize in *The Impatient Woman's Guide*.

Taking Charge of Your Fertility by Toni Weschler. This is the bible of charting; no other book even touches it in the amazing amount of detail about how to read your natural fertility signs. If you've decided you want to chart (take your temperature and check cervical mucus), buy this book. You cannot Google most of what's here, so you need the book. Weschler not only teaches you what you need to know but also makes a very convincing case for why every woman should learn to chart. The techniques in the book are backed up by good research, too—with three exceptions: First, it assumes that the day of ovulation is the most fertile, which it's not. Second, it advises sex only every other day for men with low sperm count, while recent research has shown that abstinence doesn't increase fertility. Third, the chapter on choosing the sex of your baby is based on the Shettles method and not on the research studies showing that the opposite timing actually works better.

Preventing Miscarriage by Dr. John Scher and Carol Dix. Written by a doctor who specializes in helping women stay pregnant, this book has both good information and the sensitivity necessary for this topic. Women's stories are woven throughout, and the emotional side of miscarriage is mentioned often, as it should be. The book explains why miscarriages occur and what can be done about repeat miscarriages. The doctor is an advocate of IVG, a blood product sometimes used after repeat miscarriages that's somewhat controversial, but that's the only part of the book that's unusual.

Inconceivable by Julia Indichova. Julia was 42 when she started trying to get pregnant with her second child and discovered she had high FSH. This slim volume is her story of seeing a slate of fertility doctors, Chinese medicine practitioners, and anyone else who could offer even a remote chance of helping her get pregnant. In the end, she improved her diet, maintained her optimism, and got pregnant naturally. It's a well-told story and great for finding inspiration if you're struggling with fertility issues and/or are older. Julia really captures the pain of infertility, especially when you're older and doctors tell you there is nothing they can do. This is definitely a personal story rather than anything based on research, so read it in that way. (In other words, don't go out and start drinking wheatgrass juice by the gallon.)

Three Wishes by Carey Goldberg, Beth Jones, and Pamela Ferdinand. This triple memoir is the story of three women, all in their late 30s, who wanted to be mothers and decided to use a sperm donor. Carey bought the sperm first, then passed it on to Beth, who then passed it on to Pam. I won't tell you why they kept playing pass the sperm, because that would ruin your enjoyment of the stories. They're good ones, with as many plot twists as a good novel.

The Depression Cure by Steve Ilardi, Ph.D. Even if you've never been depressed, you should read this book. Dr. Ilardi's natural mood boosters (like omega-3s, sunshine, and exercise) can help almost anyone feel better. The book is easy and fun to read and even has a troubleshooting section. Dr. Ilardi's advice is very specific and will inspire you to live better and thus feel better.

References

Here are the scientific studies I used in the book. You should be able to find the abstract (a short summary) of the articles online for free. The full articles are accessible at university libraries or online for a fee; you might be able to find a few online for free. To search for new articles on a topic, use the database Medline.

Chapter 1: What to Do Before You Start Trying

Barad, D., & Gleicher, N. (2006). Effect of dehydroepiandrosterone on oocyte and embryo yields, embryo grade and cell number in IVF. *Human Reproduction, 21,* 2845–2849.

Barad, D., Brill, H., & Gleicher, N. (2007). Update on the use of dehydroepiandrosterone supplementation among women with diminished ovarian function. *Journal of Assisted Reproductive Genetics, 24,* 629–634.

Battaglia, C. et al. (2002). Adjuvant L-arginine treatment in controlled ovarian hyperstimulation: A double-blind, randomized study. *Human Reproduction, 17,* 659–665.

Boivin, J., Griffiths, E., & Venetis, C. A. (2011). Emotional distress in infertile women and failure of assisted reproductive technologies: Meta-analysis of prospective psychosocial studies. *British Medical Journal 342,* d223.

Caan, B., Quesenberry, C. P., & Coates, A. O. (1998). Differences in fertility associated with caffeinated beverage consumption. *American Journal of Public Health, 88,* 270–274.

Cheong, Y. et al. (2010). Acupuncture and herbal medicine in in vitro fertilization: A review of the evidence for clinical practice. *Human Fertility, 13,* 3–12.

Dennehy, C. E. (2006). The use of herbs and dietary supplements in gynecology: An evidence-based review. *Journal of Midwifery & Women's Health, 51,* 402–409.

Domar, A. D. et al. (2009). The impact of acupuncture on in vitro fertilization outcome. *Fertility and Sterility, 91,* 723–726.

Domar, A. D. et al. (2010). The relationship between stress and IVF outcome. *Fertility and Sterility, 94,* S66.

Fujimoto, V. Y. et al. (2011). Serum unconjugated bisphenol A concentrations in women may adversely influence oocyte quality during in vitro fertilization. *Fertility and Sterility, 95,* 1816–1819.

Gijsen, V. et al. (2008). Does light drinking during pregnancy improve pregnancy outcome? A critical commentary. *Canadian Journal of Clinical Pharmacology, 15,* e782–e786.

Gleicher, N. et al. (2009). Miscarriage rates after dehydroepiandrosterone (DHEA) supplementation in women with diminished ovarian reserve: A case control study. *Reproductive Biology and Endocrinology, 7,* 108.

Gleicher, N., Weghofer, A., & Barad, D. H. (2010). Dehydroepiandrosterone (DHEA) reduces embryo aneuploidy: Direct evidence from preimplantation genetic screening (PGS). *Reproductive Biology and Endocrinology, 8,* 140.

Gleicher, N., Weghofer, A., & Barad, D. H. (2010). Improvement in diminished ovarian reserve after dehydroepiandrosterone supplementation. *Reproductive BioMedicine Online, 21,* 360–365.

Gnoth, C. et al. (2003). Time to pregnancy: Results of the German prospective study and impact on the management of infertility. *Human Reproduction, 18,* 1959–1966.

Hakim, R. B., Gray, R. H., & Zacur, H. (1998). Alcohol and caffeine consumption and decreased fertility. *Fertility and Sterility, 70,* 6329–6370.

Hilgers, T. W. et al. (1992). Cumulative pregnancy rates in patients with apparently normal fertility and fertility-focused intercourse. *Journal of Reproductive Medicine, 37*, 864.

Jensen, T. K. et al. (1998). Caffeine intake and fecundability: A follow-up study among 430 Danish couples planning their first pregnancy. *Reproductive Toxicology, 12*, 289–295.

Mamas, L., & Mamas, E. (2009). Premature ovarian failure and dehydroepiandrosterone. *Fertility and Sterility, 91*, 644–646.

Milewicz, A. et al. (1993). Vitex angus castus extract in the treatment of luteal phase defects due to latent hyperprolactinema: Results of a randomized placebo-controlled double-blind study. *Arzeimittel-Forschung, 43*, 752–756.

Moy, I. et al. (2011). Randomized controlled trial: Effects of acupuncture on pregnancy rates in women undergoing in vitro fertilization. *Fertility and Sterility, 95*, 583–587.

Practice Committee of the American Society for Reproductive Medicine. (2008). Optimizing natural fertility. *Fertility and Sterility, 90*, S1–S6.

Roseboom, T. J. et al. (2001). Effects of prenatal exposure to the Dutch famine on adult disease in later life: An overview. *Molecular and Cellular Endocrinology, 185*, 93–98.

Seckl, J. R. (2001). Glucocorticoid programming of the fetus: Adult phenotypes and molecular mechanisms. *Molecular and Cellular Endocrinology, 185*, 61–71.

Sonmezer, M. et al. (2009). Dehydroepiandrosterone supplementation improves ovarian response and cycle outcome in poor responders. *Reproductive BioMedicine Online, 19*, 508–513.

Westphal, L. M., Plan, M. L., & Trant, A. S. (2006). Double-blind, placebo-controlled study of FertilityBlend: A nutritional supplement for improving fertility in women. *Clinical and Experimental Obstetrics & Gynecology, 33*, 2050–208.

Whelan, A. M., Jurgens, T. M., & Naylor, H. (2009). Herbs, vitamins and minerals in the treatment of premenstrual syndrome: A systematic review. *Canadian Journal of Clinical Pharmacology, 16,* e430–e431.

Wiser, A. et al. (2010). Addition of dehydroepiandrosterone (DHEA) for poor-responder patients before and during IVF treatment improves the pregnancy rate: A randomized prospective study. *Human Reproduction, 25,* 2496–2500.

Zhu, B.-P. et al. (2001). Effect of the interval between pregnancies on perinatal outcomes among white and black women. *American Journal of Obstetrics and Gynecology, 185,* 1403–1410.

Chapter 2: Supplements, Exercise, and the SOS Diet

Bouchard, M. F. et al. (2010). Attention-deficit/hyperactivity disorder and urinary metabolities of organophosphate pesticides. *Pediatrics, 125,* e1270–e1277.

Buck Louis, G. M. et al. (2009). Polychlorinated biphenyl serum concentrations, lifestyle, and time-to-pregnancy. *Human Reproduction, 24,* 451–458.

Chavarro, J. E. et al. (2007). Diet and lifestyle in the prevention of ovulatory disorder infertility. *Obstetrics & Gynecology, 110,* 1050–1058.

Chavarro, J. E. et al. (2007). Dietary fatty acid intakes and the risk of ovulatory infertility. *The American Journal of Clinical Nutrition, 85,* 231–237.

Chavarro, J. E. et al. (2006). Iron intake and risk of ovulatory infertility. *Obstetrics & Gynecology, 108,* 1145–1152.

Czeizel, A. E., Metneki, J., & Dudas, I. (1996). The effect of preconceptional multivitamin supplementation on fertility. *International Journal of Vitamin and Nutrition Research, 66,* 55–58.

Hammiche, F. et al. (2011). Increased preconception omega-3 ployunsaturated fatty acid intake improves embryo morphology. *Fertility and Sterility, 95,* 1820–1823.

Hassan, M. A. M., & Killick, S. R. (2004). Negative lifestyle is associated with a significant reduction in fecundity. *Fertility and Sterility, 81,* 384–392.

Jacobson, J. L. et al. (2008). Beneficial effects of a polyunsaturated fatty acid on infant development: Evidence from the Inuit of arctic Quebec. *Journal of Pediatrics, 152,* 356–364.

Jacques, C. et al. (2011). Long-term effects of prenatal omega-3 fatty acid intake on visual function in school-age children. *Journal of Pediatrics, 158,* 83–90.

Lim, S. S., Noakes, M., & Norman, R. J. (2007). Dietary effects on fertility treatment and pregnancy outcomes. *Current Opinion in Endocrinology, Diabetes, & Obesity, 14,* 465–469.

Seibel, M. M. (1999). The role of nutrition and nutritional supplements in women's health. *Fertility and Sterility, 72,* 579–591.

Vujkovic, M. et al. (2010). The preconception Mediterranean dietary pattern in couples undergoing in vitro fertilization: Intracyctoplasmic sperm injection treatment increases the chance of pregnancy. *Fertility and Sterility, 94,* 2096–2101.

Williams, N. I. et al. (1999). Effects of short-term strenuous endurance exercise upon corpus luteum function. *Medicine and Science in Sports and Exercise, 31,* 949–958.

Chapter 3: Not the Kind of Egg That Comes in a Carton: How to Figure Out When You Are Ovulating

Bigelow, J. L. et al. (2004). Mucus observations in the fertile window: A better predictor of conception than timing of intercourse. *Human Reproduction, 19,* 889–892.

Fehring, R. J., Raviele, K., & Schneider, M. (2004). A comparison of the fertile phase as determined by the ClearPlan Easy Fertility Monitor and self-assessment of cervical mucus. *Contraception, 69,* 9–14.

Scarpa, B., Dunson, D. B., & Giacchi, E. (2007). Bayesian selection of optimal rules for timing intercourse to conceive by using calendar and mucus. *Fertility and Sterility, 88,* 915–924.

Scolaro, K. L., Lloyd, K. B., & Helms, K. L. (2008). Devices for home evaluation of women's health concerns. *American Journal of Health-System Pharmacy, 65*, 299–314.

Tanabe, K., et al. (2001). Prediction of the potentially fertile period by urinary hormone measurements using a new home-use monitor: Comparison with laboratory hormone analyses. *Human Reproduction, 16*, 1619–1624.

Chapter 4: Horizontal Mambo: The Best Time to Dance the Baby Dance

Barrett, J. C., & Marshall, J. (1967). The risk of conception on different days of the menstrual cycle. *Population Studies, 23*, 455.

Behre, H. M. et al. (2000). Prediction of ovulation by urinary hormone measurements with the home use ClearPlan Fertility Monitor: Comparison with transvaginal ultrasound scans and serum hormone measurements. *Human Reproduction, 15*, 2478–2482.

Check, J. H., Epstein, R., & Long, R. (1995). Effect of time interval between ejaculations on semen parameters. *Archives of Andrology, 27*, 93–95.

Colombo, B., & Masarotto, G. (2000). Daily fecundability: First results from a new database. *Demographic Research, 3*, 5.

Custers, I. M. et al. (2009). Immobilisation versus immediate mobilisation after intrauterine insemination. *British Medical Journal, 339*, b4080.

Dunson, D. B. et al. (2001). Assessing human fertility using several markers of ovulation. *Statistics in Medicine, 20*, 965–978.

Dunson, D. B. et al. (1999). Day-specific probabilities of clinical pregnancy based on two studies with imperfect measures of ovulation. *Human Reproduction, 14*, 1835–1839.

Dunson, D. B., Colombo, B., & Baird, D. D. (2002). Changes with age in the level and duration of fertility in the menstrual cycle. *Human Reproduction, 17*, 1399–1403.

Kunz, G. et al. (1996). The dynamics of rapid sperm transport through the female genital tract: Evidence from vaginal sonography of uterine peristalsis and hysterosalpingoscintigraphy. *Human Reproduction, 11,* 627–632.

Levitas, E. et al. (2005). Relationship between the duration of sexual abstinence and semen quality: Analysis of 9,489 semen samples. *Fertility and Sterility, 83,* 1680–1686.

Munkelwitz, R., & Gilbert, B. R. (1998). Are boxer shorts really better? A critical analysis of the role of underwear type in male subfertility. *Journal of Urology, 160,* 1329–1333.

Stanford, J. B., & Dunson, D. B. (2007). Effects of sexual intercourse patterns in time to pregnancy studies. *American Journal of Epidemiology, 165,* 1088–1095.

Stanford, J. B., White, G. L., & Hatasaka, H. (2002). Timing intercourse to achieve pregnancy: Current evidence. *Obstetrics & Gynecology, 100,* 1333–1341.

Wilcox, A. J., Weinberg, C. R., & Baird, D. D. (1998). Post-ovulatory ageing of the human oocyte and embryo failure. *Human Reproduction, 13,* 394–397.

Chapter 5: Choosing the Sex of Your Baby

France, J. T. et al. (1992). Characteristics of natural conceptual cycles occurring in a prospective study of sex preselection: Fertility awareness symptoms, hormone levels, sperm survival, and pregnancy outcome. *International Journal of Fertility, 37,* 244–255.

France, J. T. et al. (1984). A prospective study of the preselection of the sex of offspring by timing intercourse relative to ovulation. *Fertility and Sterility, 41,* 894.

Gray, R. H. (1991). Natural family planning and sex selection: Fact or fiction? *American Journal of Obstetrics and Gynecology, 165,* 1982–1984.

Gray, R. H. et al. (1998). Sex ratio associated with timing of insemination and length of the follicular phase in planned and unplanned pregnancies during use of natural family planning. *Human Reproduction, 13,* 1397–1400.

Guerrero, R. (1974). Association of the type and time of insemination within the menstrual cycle with the human sex ratio at birth. *New England Journal of Medicine, 291,* 1056–1059.

Mathews, F. et al. (2008). You are what your mother eats: Evidence for maternal preconception diet influencing foetal sex in humans. *Proceedings of the Royal Society B (Biological Sciences), 275,* 1661–1668.

Perez, A. et al. (1985). Sex ratio associated with natural family planning. *Fertility and Sterility, 43,* 152–153.

Ryan, E. A. J. et al. (2008). The sex ratio of offspring born to women, using dehydroepiandrosterone (DHEA) to improve ovarian response. *Fertility and Sterility, 90,* S116–S117.

Shettles, L. B. (1974). Factors influencing sex ratios. *International Journal of Gynaecology and Obstetrics, 8,* 643–647.

Simcock, B. W. (1985). Sons and daughters—a sex preselection study. *Medical Journal of Australia, 142,* 541–542.

Stolkowski, J., & Lorrain, J. (1980). Preconceptual selection of fetal sex. *International Journal of Gynaecology and Obstetrics, 18,* 440–443.

Wilcox, A. J., Weinberg, C. R., & Baird, D. D. (1995). Timing of sexual intercourse in relation to ovulation—effects on the probability of conception, survival of the pregnancy, and sex of the baby. *New England Journal of Medicine, 333,* 1517–1521.

World Health Organization. (1984). A prospective multicentre study of the ovulation method of natural family planning: IV. The outcome of pregnancy. *Fertility and Sterility, 41,* 593–598.

Zarutskie, P. W. et al. (1989). The clinical relevance of sex selection techniques. *Fertility and Sterility, 52,* 891–905.

References

Chapter 6: Not as Scary as You've Heard: The Real Stats on Age and Fertility

American Society for Reproductive Medicine. (2003). *Age and Fertility: A Guide for Patients.*

Belloc, S. (2008). Effect of maternal and paternal age on pregnancy and miscarriage rates after intrauterine insemination. *Reproductive BioMedicine Online, 17,* 392–397.

Dunson, D. B., Baird, D. D., & Colombo, B. (2004). Increased infertility with age in men and women. *American Journal of Obstetrics and Gynecology, 103,* 51–56.

Dunson, D. B., Colombo, B. & Baird, D. D. (2002). Changes with age in the level and duration of fertility in the menstrual cycle. *Human Reproduction, 17,* 1399–1403.

Hassan, M. A. M., & Killick, S. R. (2003). Effect of male age on fertility: Evidence for the decline in male fertility with increasing age. *Fertility and Sterility, 79,* 1520–1527.

Heffner, L. J. (2004). Advanced maternal age—how old is too old? *New England Journal of Medicine, 351,* 1927–1930.

Jansen, R. P. S. (2003). The effect of female age on the likelihood of a live birth from one in-vitro fertilization treatment. *Medical Journal of Australia, 178,* 258–261.

Klipstein, S. et al. (2005). One last chance for pregnancy: A review of 2,705 in vitro fertilization cycles initiated in women age 40 years and above. *Fertility and Sterility, 84,* 435–445.

Leridon, H. (2004). Can assisted reproduction technology compensate for the natural decline in fertility with age? A model assessment. *Human Reproduction, 19,* 1548–1553.

Maseelall, P. B., & McGovern, P. G. (2008). Ovarian reserve screening: What the general gynecologist should know. *Women's Health, 4,* 291–300.

Menken, J., Trussell, J., & Larsen, U. (1986). Age and infertility. *Science, 26,* 1389–1394.

Nikolaou, D., & Templeton, A. (2004). Early ovarian ageing. *Euro-*

pean Journal of Obstetrics, Gynecology, and Reproductive Biology, 113, 126–133.

Sills, E. S., Alper, M. M., & Walsh, A. P. H. (2009). Ovarian reserve screening in infertility: Practical applications and theoretical directions for research. *European Journal of Obstetrics, Gynecology, and Reproductive Biology, 146*, 30–36.

Chapter 7: "If One More Person Tells Me to 'Just Relax' . . .": The Psychological Side of Getting Pregnant

Cousineau, T. M., & Domar, A. D. (2007). Psychological impact of infertility. *Clinical Obstetrics & Gynecology, 21*, 293–308.

Domar, A. D. (2000). Impact of group psychological interventions on pregnancy rates in infertile women. *Fertility and Sterility, 73*, 805–811.

Francis, M. E., & Pennebaker, J. W. (1992). Putting stress into words: The impact of writing on physiological absentee, and self-reported emotional well-being measures. *American Journal of Health Promotion, 6*, 280–287.

Friedler, S. et al. (2011). The effect of medical cloning on pregnancy rates after in vitro fertilization and embryo transfer (IVF-ET). *Fertility and Sterility, 95*, 2127–2130.

Ilardi, S. S. (2009). *The Depression Cure: The 6-Step Program to Beat Depression Without Drugs.* Cambridge, MA: Da Capo Press.

Lambert, N. M. et al. (2009). A changed perspective: How gratitude can affect sense of coherence through positive reframing. *Journal of Positive Psychology, 4*, 461–470.

Nolen-Hoeksema, S., Wisco, B. E., & Lyubomirsky, S. (2008). Rethinking rumination. *Perspectives on Psychological Science, 3*, 400–424.

Norem, J. K., & Cantor, N. (1986). Defensive pessimism: Harnessing anxiety as motivation. *Journal of Personality and Social Psychology, 51*, 1208–1217.

Norem, J. K., & Chang, E. C. (2002). The positive psychology of negative thinking. *Journal of Clinical Psychology, 58*, 993–1001.

Pennebaker, J. W., & O'Heeron, R. C. (1984). Confiding in others and illness rate among spouses of suicide and accidental death victims. *Journal of Abnormal Psychology, 93,* 473–476.

Rood, L. et al. (2009). The influence of emotion-focused rumination and distraction on depressive symptoms in non-clinical youth. *Clinical Psychology Review, 29,* 607–616.

Twenge, J. M., Baumeister, R. F., DeWall, C. N., Ciarocco, N. J., & Bartels, J. M. (2007). Social exclusion decreases prosocial behavior. *Journal of Personality and Social Psychology, 92,* 56–66.

Twenge, J. M., Baumeister, R. F., Tice, D. M., & Stucke, T. S. (2001). If you can't join them, beat them: Effects of social exclusion on aggressive behavior. *Journal of Personality and Social Psychology, 81,* 1058–1069.

Twenge, J. M., Catanese, K. R., & Baumeister, R. F. (2002). Social exclusion causes self-defeating behavior. *Journal of Personality and Social Psychology, 83,* 606–615.

Chapter 8: Peeing on More Sticks: The Two-Week Wait and When to Test for Pregnancy

Sayle, A. E. et al. (2002). A prospective study of the onset of symptoms of pregnancy. *Journal of Clinical Epidemiology, 55,* 676–680.

Wilcox, A. J. et al. (2001). Natural limits of pregnancy testing in relation to the expected menstrual period. *Journal of the American Medical Association, 286,* 1759–1761.

Wilcox, A. J., Baird, D. D., & Weinberg, C. R. (1999). Time of implantation of the conceptus and loss of pregnancy. *New England Journal of Medicine, 340,* 1796–1800.

Wilcox, A. J., Weinberg, C. R., & Baird, D. D. (1995). Timing of sexual intercourse in relation to ovulation—effects on the probability of conception, survival of the pregnancy, and sex of the baby. *New England Journal of Medicine, 333,* 1517–1521.

Chapter 9: Sad Endings: Miscarriage

Bhattacharya, S. (2011). Pregnancy following miscarriage: What is the optimum interpregnancy interval? *Women's Health, 7,* 139–141.

Leridon, H. (2008). A new estimate of permanent sterility by age: Sterility defined as the inability to conceive. *Population Studies, 62,* 15–24.

Love, E. R. et al. (2010). Effect of interpregnancy interval on outcomes of pregnancy after miscarriage: Retrospective analysis of hospital episode statistics in Scotland. *British Medical Journal, 341,* 3967.

Price, M., Kelsberg, G., & Safranek, S. (2005). What treatments prevent miscarriage after recurrent pregnancy loss? *Journal of Family Practice, 54,* 892–894.

Wnag, X. et al. (2003). Conception, early pregnancy loss, and time to clinical pregnancy: A population-based prospective study. *Fertility and Sterility, 79,* 577–584.

Chapter 10: When to See Your Doctor and What to Expect When You Do

Gnoth, C. et al. (2005). Definition and prevalence of subfertility and infertility. *Human Reproduction, 20,* 1144–1147.

Appendix G

Vear, C. S. (1977). Preselective sex determination. *Medical Journal of Australia, 2,* 700–702.

Williamson, N. E., Lean, T. H., & Vengadasalam, D. (1978). Evaluation of an unsuccessful sex preselection clinic in Singapore. *Journal of Biosocial Sciences, 10,* 375–388.

Acknowledgments

One summer day when I was six months pregnant with my second child, I was swimming laps when an idea popped into my head: Why don't I write a book called *The Impatient Woman's Guide to Getting Pregnant?* Over the previous four years, I'd read countless journal articles about fertility, worried constantly, and wished I could snap my fingers and get pregnant *right now*. I knew there were other women who felt that way, too.

I already had a call scheduled with my agent, Jill Kneerim, to discuss my ideas for my next book. I started with my Big Academic Idea, with lots of evidence (most of it depressing), and by the end of my recitation, Jill and I agreed that the ideas were solid, but it might be tough to sell. Then, as almost an afterthought, I mentioned *The Impatient Woman's Guide*, saying I wanted to write a girlfriend-to-girlfriend advice book that was fun to read. She said, "Tell me more about that one," and sure enough, here we are. So my first thanks are to Jill, for seeing the potential in the idea of a neurotic research psychologist mom writing a fertility book. Jill's assistant, Caroline Zimmerman, was also indispensible, summarizing other books in the area so that we could make it clear that this one was definitely different.

The crack editorial team of Leslie Meredith and Donna Loffredo ably guided the project from proposal to a final manuscript, catching my overuse of acronyms and my occasional bad joke. (If worse jokes remain, the fault is mine.)

My biggest debt of gratitude is to the women who shared their stories with me, either through my survey at www.jean-twenge.com or through our personal connection. Your insights brought the topic of fertility exactly where it should be: about real women and what they experience. Thanks as well to friends who referred others to the site, especially Cara Fairfax, Deborah Johnson, Nicole Kalian, Amy Tobia, and Sarah Kilabarda. Andrew Chapman and Brian Cowell provided crucial webpage design.

Four friends read chapters and provided amazing feedback and material. My sister-in-law, Amanda Louden, a certified nutrition educator, read Chapter 2 on food and kept me from making several embarrassing newbie mistakes, as well as enlightening me about whole grains, organic versus local food, and the joys of steel-cut oats. Jeff Green imparted the guy's perspective with some awesome jokes. Jody Davis and Benita Jackson helped immensely as both psychology experts and readers from the target demographic. Jeff and Jody also recommended my new favorite show, *I Didn't Know I Was Pregnant*.

Thanks to Keith Campbell for being my foxhole buddy in everything from academic debates to helicopter rides—looking forward to the next book. My eternal gratitude goes to friends who patiently listened to my irrational worries, especially Sonia Orfield and Stacy Campbell. Thanks as well to those who provided friendship and support, including Ken Bloom, Lawrence Charap, Cara Fairfax, Craig Foster, Deborah Johnson, Mike and Kelly Johnson, Darlene and Rich Kobylar, Claire Murphy, Nell Newman, Adam Shah, Susan and Alistair Steele, Amy and Paul Tobia, and May Yeh. A big hug to Rita Pandya and her family (including new mom Mona and baby Nisha) for taking such good care of Elizabeth.

My parents, Steve and JoAnn Twenge, provided crucial babysitting, lots of grandma and grandpa love, and many Sunday dinners. We are happy to have you here in paradise. All of us look forward to video visits from Grammy Susie, Papa Jud, and the chicken. Dan Tvenge, Kendel Neidermyer, and Alex Berman, thanks for coming—you can play monster with us in the pool anytime. Aunt Pat and Papa Bud, thanks for the boat rides, the tubing, and the snacks. Marilyn and Ray Swenson; Jane, Brian, and Roxanne Moening; Sarah and Dan Kilabarda; Anna, Dusty, and Henry Wetzel; and Brian, Kim, Abby, and Owen Chapeau, I love you all and always love seeing you. Thanks to Roxanne Moening for sending me our family tree, and to Mark, Kathy, and Katie Moening for the horses and for the inspiration.

My daughters are the reason I wrote this book. All of the worry and craziness of fertility happens for one big reason: We long for our children even before they are conceived. Kate and Elizabeth, you are more than worth it. Elizabeth, thank you for your enthusiastic greetings ("Hi! Hi!") and your snuggles. Kate, I am charmed every day by your joy in learning, even if I do take too long to explain some things. (Kate: "Mommy, what's reelection?" Me: Talk for about a minute, using simple words but probably still too long. Kate, the second I stop talking: "Mommy, some-times people poop in their underwear.") And thank you for being so nice to your sister. The definition of lucky: having a 4-year-old who shares her dessert with her sibling.

And to my husband, Craig, thanks for enduring my fer-tility craziness—three times—and not losing it, and then enduring a modified version when I was creating this book. An Impatient Woman needs a patient man, and I'm lucky to have found that in you.

Index

abstinence, 90, 203
acronyms, 185–86
acupuncture, 16–17, 123
adoption, 23, 131
Advanced Fertility Center, 110
age, xiii, 102–15
    birth defects and, 107–8
    miscarriages and, 106
    psychology of, 111–14
    timing of sex and, 104
alcohol, xv, 2, 3, 4–5, 9, 26,
    188, 189
allergies, 30
amazon.com, 65–66
American Society for
    Reproductive Medicine,
    103
amniocentesis, 108
anencephaly, 36
anger, 153
Angie's List, 174
antibiotics, 6, 161, 167
antidepressants, 25, 133
anti-Müllerian hormone
    (AMH), 109
antral follicles, 109, 110
anxiety, ix, x, xvi–xvii, 1, 73,
    117–18, 133, 144
    combatting, xvii, 118–33

fertility not affected by, 24,
    26, 184
aphrodisiacs, 84, 184, 191
apples, 47
Appleton, Sarah, ix–xi
arctic char, 44
"Are Boxer Shorts Really
    Better? A Critical
    Analysis of the Role of
    Underwear Type in Male
    Subfertility," 9
aromatherapy, 123
Astroglide, 82
autism, 35
avocados, 34

baby food, 48
Baby Mama (film), 130
baby showers, 132
bananas, 97
Barad, David, 20–21
basal body temperature
    (BBT), 57–58, 61,
    72–73, 185
Belkin, Lisa, 86
birth control, 1, 14, 32, 79
birth-control pills, 14, 56, 62,
    79, 187, 188, 196

birth defects, 2, 36, 107–8
    chromosomal, 21
bisphenol-A (BPA), 15, 191
blogs, 167
blood tests, 108, 169–70
blood thinners, 161
body mass index (BMI), 33,
    34, 187
bok choy, 38, 42, 48, 193
boys, choosing of, 94, 95, 96,
    97, 183
brain, 38
brain system, xv
bread, 37, 40
breakfast cereal, 95, 98, 99
breastfeeding, 71, 115, 179,
    196
    ovulation prediction while,
    73–74
breasts, 147
breathing trouble, 70
broccoli, 38
"bug" position, 83
butter, 50

caesarean sections, 70–71,
    180, 181
caffeine, 2, 3–5, 26, 189
cake, 49
calcium, 35, 48, 95, 97, 99,
    101, 190
calcium supplements, 19
calorie consumption, 95–96
carbohydrates, 37, 95
career, xiii
catfish, 45
celery, 47
Center for Human
    Reproduction (CHR), 20

cervical mucus, xiv, 54–57, 60,
    91, 200, 203
    while breastfeeding, 74
    drying of, 171–72
    eggwhite, 55–56, 64, 78,
    185, 196
    sex of baby and, 94
charting, 14, 32, 54–61, 64,
    66, 72, 73, 127, 138,
    142, 149, 166, 183, 188,
    200, 203
    while breastfeeding, 74
    and false positives on OPKs,
    69
    obsessing over, 60, 72
    after positive pregnancy
    test, 156–57
    pregnancy tests and, 142
    sex selection and, 94
    troubleshooting with, 195
chasteberry, 17
cheese, 97
chemical pregnancies, 154
    see also miscarriages
chemicals, 16
chicken, 193
chicken pox, 11
child spacing, 30–31
Chinese birth chart, 92
Chinese Gender Chart, 99–100
Chinese medicine herbs, 17
chloride levels, 67
Choosing the Sex of Your
    Baby: The Method Best
    Supported by Scientific
    Evidence (Shettles and
    Rorvik), 198–99
chorionic villus sampling
    (CVS), 108

chromosomal birth defects, 21
clams, 45
Clearblue Easy fertility
    monitor, 63, 64, 65–67,
    78, 79, 190
ClearPlan Easy Ovulation Test
    Pack, 62
Clomid, 71, 87, 171–72, 174,
    175, 195
cod, 44
coffee, 3–4
Coleman, Joshua, 85
collard greens, 48
conception, timing of, x
Conception Chronicles, The
    (Debano), 57, 81, 130
condoms, 14, 79
Conquering Infertility (Domar),
    124
Consumer Reports, 62, 143
Copperman, Alan, 86
CoQ-10 supplements, 22–23,
    190
Costco, 190
cough syrup, 57
cowgirl position, 83

dairy, 47–48
dating, 129, 135
David, Sami, 172–73
Debano, Patty, 56–57, 81
deep breathing, xvii, 122–23,
    180
defensive pessimism, 128–30
dehydroepiandrosterone
    (DHEA) supplements,
    20–22, 98, 190
dental offices, 16
dental problems, 12

dentists, 188
DepoProvera, 14, 187
depression, 26, 128
    antidepressants and, 133
    combatting, xvii, 36, 121,
        184
    fertility affected by, 25, 117
    infertility and, 125
    rumination as cause of, 119,
        184
    symptoms of, 124
Depression Cure, The (Ilardi),
    121, 204
DHA, 36
DHEA supplements, 20–22,
    98, 190
diabetes, 13
diet, x, 1, 33–51, 92, 96, 157,
    190–91, 192–94
    and choosing sex of baby,
        95–99
    fatty, 48
    Mediterranean, 43, 183
    SOS, 39–40, 44, 183
    see also specific foods
diminished ovarian reserve,
    109–10
diphtheria, 11, 188
direct coombs, 170
disordered testicular
    thermoregulation, 9
distractions, 119
Dix, Carol, 203–4
doctors, 165
    preconception visits to,
        11–14, 187
doggy style, 83
Domar, Alice, 24, 25, 123–24,
    172

douching, 90, 92, 100
doula, 179–80
Down syndrome, 21, 107, 108, 115
Dratch, Rachel, 113
drugs, 9, 188
drugstore.com, 17, 65–66
DTaP (diphtheria, tetanus, and pertussis), 11, 188

early loss, 154
　　see also miscarriages
eggs:
　　aging of, 105
　　life span of, 52–53, 76
　　number of, 112, 114
　　weak, 71
eggwhites, 82
embryos, 91
　　chromosomal mistakes in, 107
　　implantation of, 3
environmental hazards, 15–16
envy, 137–39
EPA, 36, 121
epidural, 180
Epsom salt baths, 123
erythromycin, 161
estrogen, 63
evening primrose oil, 18
exercise, x, 33, 34, 50–51, 71, 188
　　to boost mood, 121–22

Facebook, 132
faith, 131–32
fallopian tubes, 84, 109, 170, 171, 174, 197

fat, 34, 48
fatigue, 29–30
Feeling Good, 25
Ferdinand, Pamela, 204
FertiBella, 18–19
fertility:
　　as affected by depression, 25, 117
　　age limit to, 114–15
　　anxiety created by, 118
　　high, *see* high fertility
　　husbands' ignorance of, 80
　　peak, *see* peak fertility
　　psychology of, 111–14
　　treatment for, 165–76; *see also specific treatment*
　　see also pregnancy
Fertility Blend, 17, 18, 19, 22
Fertility Diet, The, 39, 40, 43–44, 48, 50
fertility doctors, xiv
FertilityFriend.com, 59, 78, 142, 149
fertility monitors, 32, 54, 63–68, 80, 81, 106, 118, 122, 127, 138, 162, 166, 183, 188, 195, 196
　　anxiety over, 73
　　while breastfeeding, 74
　　Clearblue Easy, 63, 64, 65–67, 78, 79, 190
　　false positives on, 163
　　obsessing over, 72
　　pregnancy tests and, 142
　　reading of, 64–65
　　sex of baby and, 94
　　used, 65, 66–67
fertility signs, 28

fertility tests, 19, 171, 196
    see also specific tests
Fey, Tina, 111, 113
fiber, 41
fibroids, 161, 168, 197
First Response Early Result,
    143
First Response Fertility Test,
    109
Fisch, Harry, 8
fish, 38, 43–46, 183, 193
fish oil, xvii
flaxseed oil, 36
flounder, 44, 45
flow cytometer, 86
folate, 2, 35, 36, 43, 95
follicle-stimulating hormone
    (FSH), 22, 109, 169–70,
    185, 204
food, xv, 26
Food and Drug
    Administration, 45
Foreman grill, 46, 193
foreplay, 82
France, 103, 115, 184
France, John, 200
free time, 178
friends, 121, 132
frosting, 49
fruit, 47

garlic powder, 193
Genetics and IVF Institute, 86
GenSelect, 100
Gerber's Banana and Mixed
    Berries, 48
German measles, 11
ginger juice, 190
girlfriends, 28

girls, choosing of, 94–96, 183
Gleicher, Norbert, 20, 21
God, 131–32, 136, 159
Goldberg, Carey, 106–7,
    111–12, 148, 163, 204
grains, 47
gratitude, 120–21
grief, 159
grilled chicken, 193
grilled fish, 193
gum infections, 12

habitual aborters, 159
halibut, 45
Harben, Dwyn, 20
Hashimoto's thyroiditis, 12
health insurance, 5, 187
heart, 2, 38
heart disease, 36
heparin, 161
herbs, 17–18, 19
herring, 44, 45
Hewlett, Sylvia, 111
high fertility, 63–64, 73, 79
    sex of baby and, 94
home monitoring kits, x
hormonal birth control, 14
hot tubs, 123, 188
*How to Choose the Sex of Your
    Baby* (Shettles), 89–90
human chorionic
    gonadotropin (HCG),
    141, 143, 145, 155, 163,
    185
Human Reproduction, 103
humor, 130
hunger, 37
husband, fertility of, 4
    see also semen, analysis of

husbands, xiv, 133–35
  bad lifestyle habits of, 5
  and desire for boys, 85
  ignorance of fertility by,
    80
  pregnancy tests and,
    146–47
  underwear for, 9–10
  see also semen
hypothyroidism, 197
hysterosalpingogram (HSG),
    170, 186

I Didn't Know I Was Pregnant
    (TV show), xiv, 34, 145,
    150
Ilardi, Steve, 121, 204
immunizations, 11, 188
Inconceivable (Indichova),
    138–39, 175
Indichova, Julie, 138–39, 175
induction, 180
infections, 6, 187
infertility, 125
  causes of, 5–9, 11–14,
    169–73, 195–97
  depression and, 125
  laughing about, 130
  ovulatory, 39, 40, 49, 51
  secondary, 137–39
  stress and, 24, 25, 26, 166,
    184
infertility tests, 6
intelligence, of child, xv
Internet, 148, 151
  incorrect information on,
    xiv, 19, 99–101, 140–41
  see also online message
    boards

intrauterine device (IUD), 14,
    186
intrauterine insemination
    (IUI), 25, 127, 168, 175,
    176, 197
  lying down after, 83
  in MicroSort, 86, 87
  sex selection and, 86, 87
  sperm problems helped
    by, 6
intravenous immunoglobin,
    161
in vitro fertilization (IVF),
    xvii–xix, 15, 16, 20, 21,
    24, 105, 127, 130, 144,
    173, 175, 186, 197
  expense of, 168, 172, 173
  in MicroSort, 86, 87
  multiple births with, 168
  omega-3's and, 36
iron, 36, 95
IVG, 204

jogging, 51
Jones, Beth, 204
journal, 120
Journal of General Medicine,
    100
Journal of Obstetrics &
    Gynecology and
    Reproductive Biology,
    19
Journal of Urology, 9
junk food, 34, 37, 40

kale, 48
king mackerel, 44, 45
Kirkland, 190
K-Y jelly, 82

labor, pain of, 179–80
laboratories, 16
labor coaches, 179–80
L-arginine, 17, 18
leafy green vegetables, 97, 183
legs, elevation of, 83
legumes, 43
lifestyle factors, 4–5
Lots of Sex Plan, 53–54, 77, 167
low birth weight, 30
low-dose aspirin, 161
lubricants, 57, 82, 172, 191
lupus, 161
luteal phase, 17–18, 142, 186
    tracking ovulation and, 71
    variation in, 53
luteal phase, short, 17–18, 50, 71–73
    while breastfeeding, 74
    troubleshooting with, 196
luteinizing hormone (LH), 59, 61–62, 63, 64, 91, 163, 195, 200

magnesium, 97
mahi mahi, 44
Making Babies (David), 172–73
Male Biological Clock, The (Fisch), 8
male factor, *see* semen
margarine, 49–50
massage, 123
maternity leave, 29, 187
medical journals, 113–14, 200
medical offices, 16
Medical World News, 201

meditation, 122–23
Mediterranean diet, 43, 183
Medline, 19, 100, 201
menopause, 3, 109
menstrual cycle, 142, 195
    breastfeeding and, 73–74
    irregular, 138, 171, 195
    myth of regularity of, 53, 54
    see also ovulation; periods
mercury, 16, 38, 44–45, 173, 183
meta-analyses, 89–90, 200–201
MicroSort, 86–87, 97, 198
milk, 34, 47, 97, 98
minis, 123
miscarriages, 2, 30, 106, 125, 126, 131, 153–64, 186, 203–4
    causes of, 160–62
    as common, 153
    dealing with, 157–60
    early, 145–46
    indications of, 61
    as more likely with male embryos, 91
    reactions to, 158
    and sex on day of ovulation, 77, 157
    signs of, 155–56
missionary position, 82–83
MMR (measles, mumps, rubella), 11
moms, 27
mood boosters, 121–22
morning sickness, 177, 190
Mucinex, 57, 172, 196
multivitamins, 9, 188

natural childbirth techniques,
180
nausea, 29, 30, 37, 178
negative thoughts, 123–24
nervous system, xv, 2
neural tube birth defects, 2
Newsweek, 112
New York Times Magazine, 86
New Zealand study, 90–91,
92–93, 95, 200
Nikolaou, Dimitrios, 110
Nolen-Hoeksema, Susan,
119–20
Norem, Julie, 128
North Carolina study, 92, 141,
145–46
nucheal translucency, 108
nuts, 34

OB-GYNs, 70
for infertility treatment,
169, 173–74
seeing in advance, 166
obsessiveness, 26
occult blood, 170
olive oil, 43, 193
olives, 39, 183
omega-3 fatty acids, 36, 43,
44, 121, 183, 190
online discussion groups, 28
online message boards,
126–28, 174
orange juice, 48
oranges, 97
Orenstein, Peggy, 173
organic food, 46–47
orgasm, 83
ovaries, 113
low reserve of, 109–10

overweight, 33, 34, 187
ovulation, xviii, 1, 31, 141,
186
delaying of, 23, 24
fatty diets and, 48
lack of, 171
myth of regularity of, 53,
69–70
one to two days preceding,
as best for sex, 76, 183
sex of baby and, 89, 90,
91, 93, 94–95, 183–84,
198–202
sex on day of, 76–77, 94
sweets and, 49
tracking, 2
troubleshooting with, 195
see also luteal phase
ovulation, prediction of, 23,
24, 28, 31–32, 52–74,
77–78, 140
while breastfeeding, 73–74
as cause of stress, 167
cervical mucus and, 54–57,
60, 64, 74, 78, 91
combined methods of,
68–69
fertility monitors and, *see*
fertility monitors
LH and, 59, 61–62, 63, 64,
91
miscarriages avoided by, 77,
157
temperature and, 54,
57–59, 61, 72–73, 91
ovulation predictor kits
(OPKs), xiv–xv, 32,
54, 57, 59, 61–63, 66,
130, 138, 144, 152, 162,

183, 184, 186, 188, 191, 195
anxiety over, 73
while breastfeeding, 74
false positives on, 68–69, 163
obsessiveness and, 72
pregnancy tests and, 142
reading of, 62–63
sex selection and, 94
and timing of sex, 78, 80, 81
ovulatory infertility, 39, 40, 49, 51
OV watch, 67–68
oysters, 44

Paltrow, Gwyneth, 37
panic attacks, 122
partially hydrogenated oils, 49
patch, 14
Paxil, 133
peaches, 47
peak fertility, 63, 64, 69, 73, 78–79, 152
sex selection and, 94
peanut butter, 49–50
pears, 47
People, 113
periods, 134, 142, 150–51, 185, 186
irregular, 12–13, 17, 18
symptoms of, 148
see also luteal phase
pertussis, 11, 188
pillows, 83
pizza, 40, 42
placenta, 29–30
Plan Ahead test, 109, 110
plastic wrap, 15

PMS symptoms, 18, 35
Poehler, Amy, 113
Pollan, Michael, 40
pollock, 45
polychlorinated biphenyl (PCB), 44
polycystic ovarian syndrome (PCOS), 13, 186
Positive Power of Negative Thinking, The (Norem), 128
potassium, 95, 96, 97, 99, 101
potassium gluconate, 97
potatoes, 97
poultry, 47
preconception counseling, x–xi
preconception diet, *see* diet
pregnancy:
emotional aspects of, xv
news of, 27–28
obsessing over, 6, 72–73
over 30, 108–9
over 35, 102, 103–5, 172, 184, 196
over 40, 105–7, 112, 172
planning timing of, 29–32
psychology of, 26, 116–39
sexual positions and, 82–83
signs of, 147–48
symptoms of, 1, 61, 177–78
see also fertility
pregnancy tests, xiv, 3, 122, 130, 140, 144, 171, 185
days past ovulation (DPO) to use, 140–42, 184
digital, 146–47, 151, 191
false negatives on, 142–43, 184

pregnancy tests (*cont.*)
"naked," 143–44
wait for, 148–52
preimplantation genetic
diagnosis (PGD), 86, 87
prenatal screening tests, 108
prenatal vitamins, x, 2, 35–36,
183, 190
prescription drugs, 2, 187
PreSeed lubricant, 57, 82, 171,
191, 196
Preventing Miscarriage (Scher
and Dix), 203–4
probiotics, 190
progesterone, 57, 71, 130, 149
progesterone supplements,
161–62
prolactin, 169
protein, 43, 95
ProXeed, 171
Prozac, 133
pumping, 74

quinoa, 41, 42

rainbow babies, 164
Rainbow Light's Complete
Prenatal System, 190
rast burp, 170
relationships, 118
Relaxation Response, The, 25
relaxation techniques, 122–23,
124
reproductive endocrinologists
(REs), 60, 174, 175–76,
186
Resolve, 176
rice, 192
rice milk, 48

ring, 14
Rorvik, David, 89, 198–99,
200, 202
rubella, 11, 187
rumination, 119–20, 121,
184
pattern, 14
running, 51

salmon, 34, 39, 44, 45, 46, 183
salmonella, 82
salt, 193
Saturday Night Live, 111,
112–13
scallops, 44, 45
scented oils, 82
Scher, John, 203–4
sea bass, 44
secondary infertility, 137–39
second children, 179
seeds, 34
semen:
analysis of, 5–9, 170, 171,
188, 197
bacteria in, 6
bad days for, 8–9
sex, 28, 118, 133, 178, 185
on days with eggwhite
mucus, 56
on demand, 80–82
enjoyment of, 80
legs in air after, xiii–xiv, 83
positions for, 82–84
sex, timing of, 32, 69, 75–84,
140, 165, 189, 196
age and, 104
gender of baby and, 89,
90–92, 93, 94–95, 98,
198–202

one to two days before
ovulation, 76, 183
spacing of, 77
Sex and the City (film), 150,
163–64
sex of baby, choosing, xv, xvii,
85–101
for boys, 94, 95, 96, 97, 183
chances of, 86, 87, 89, 90
cost of, 87
diet and, 95–99
for girls, 94–96, 183
natural methods of, 88–92
ovulation and, 89, 90, 91,
93, 94–95
studies on, *see* studies on
choosing sex of baby
timing of sex and, 89,
90–92, 93, 94–95, 98,
198–202
see also MicroSort;
preimplantation genetic
diagnosis (PGD)
sexual positions, 82–84
shark, 44, 45
Shettles, Landrum, 89–90, 92,
100, 183–84, 198–202,
203
shrimp, 44, 45
sleep, 26–27, 121, 124, 178
sleep deprivation, 4
sleeping pills, 30
Slow-K, 97
smells, 147
smoking, 2, 3, 4–5, 9, 188
social rejection, 117–18
sodium, 95, 97–98
sole, 44
SOS diet, 39–43, 44, 183

soy milk, 48
sperm:
cervical mucus necessary
for, 55
gender of, 89
in IUI, 86
life span of, 52
lubricants and, 82
sperm (*cont.*)
speed of, 84, 89, 91
underwear and, 9–10
sperm count, 9–10, 77, 171,
203
sperm donors, 106
spina bifida, 36
spinach, 38, 39, 97, 183, 194
spinal cord, 38
spirituality, 131–32
spit, 82
spontaneous abortion, 159
spotting, 150–51, 155
squash, 97
starches, 41
steel-cut oats, 41
stillbirths, 153
stone track, 170
"stop trying" advice, 117,
166–67
strawberries, 47
stress, x, xi, 38, 60, 116–17,
169, 170–71, 184
combatting, xvii
infertility and, 24, 25, 26,
166, 184
miscarriages caused by, 161
studies on choosing sex of
baby, 89–91, 92–93,
95–97
Australian, 90, 200

studies on choosing sex of
baby (*cont.*)
  diet and, 95–97
  meta-analyses, 89–90,
    200–201
  New Zealand, 90–91,
    92–93, 95, 200
  North Carolina, 92, 141,
    145–46
  by Shettles, 89–90, 92,
    100, 183–84, 198–202,
    203
sugar, 48
sun exposure, 4
sunlight, 4, 121
supplements, x, 16–19,
    35–36, 37, 38, 100, 127,
    196
  CoQ-10, 22–23
  DHEA, 20–22, 98
  omega-3, 36, 121, 190
  potassium, 97
  progesterone, 161–62
support groups, 124–26, 176
sweet potatoes, 193
swordfish, 44, 45

Taking Charge of Your Fertility
  (Weschler), 24, 55, 57,
    58, 203
tcoyf.com, 59
tea, 4
technetium-labeled albumin
  macrospheres of sperm
  sizes, 84
teeth, 188
temperature, 54, 57–59, 61,
    78, 138, 149, 151, 157,
    200, 203

tetanus, 11, 188
THC, 3
The Bump, 99
therapy, 125–26
Three Wishes (Goldberg, Jones
    and Ferdinand), 106,
    112, 148, 163, 204
thyroid disease, 161
thyroid hormone levels, 12,
    169
tilapia, 45
tilefish, 44, 45
Time, 113
tiredness, 178
tobacco, 2, 3, 4–5, 9
Tonglen meditation, 123
toxins, 3
Trader Joe's, 42, 190
trans fat, 49–50
trimester, first, 164, 188
  miscarriages in, 154, 162
  symptoms of, 177–78
trimester, second, as reprieve,
    178
trimester, third, 178
troubleshooting, 195–97
trout, 44
tubes, tying of, 92, 93
tuna, 45
turkey, 193–94
"Twelve-Month Pregnancy," 38
two-week wait (TWW),
    140–52

ultrasounds, 70, 79, 86, 108,
    109, 154, 164, 175
underwear, 9–10
underweight, 33, 187
Us, 113

uterine abnormalities, 161
uterine fibroids, 161, 168, 197
uterus, 24, 170

vaccinations, 11
vaginal birth, 180–81
varicoceles, 6
    surgery for, 171
vegetables, 42, 43, 47, 192,
    194
vegetable steamers, 15, 191
vegetarians, 40
Vitamin D Solution, The, 4
vitamins, xv, 9, 19, 37, 38,
    129
    A, 193
    B6, 18, 35, 36, 43, 190
    C, 188
    D, 4, 35, 97
    E zinc, 9
    folate, 2, 35, 36, 43, 95
    prenatal, x, 2, 35–36, 183,
    190
vitex, 17, 18, 22

Waiting for Daisy (Orenstein),
    173
walking, 51

warm tubs, 123
water, 82
weaning, 73, 74, 115
weight, 33
Weiner, Jennifer, 145
Wellbutrin, 133
Weschler, Toni, 24, 203
whitefish, 44
Whole Foods, 41, 42, 46
wine, 3
withdrawal, 103
woman on top position, 83
Women Who Think Too Much
    (Nolen-Hoeksema),
    119–20
working, 27
worrying, 13–14
    see also anxiety; stress

X-rays, 16
X sperm, 89, 91, 100

yoga, 122, 123
yogurt, 48, 97, 98, 192
Y sperm, 89, 91, 92, 100

0+12, 92–93
zinc, 95, 188

About the Author

Jean M. Twenge, professor of psychology at San Diego State University, is the author of more than 80 scientific publications and 2 books based on her research, *Generation Me* and *The Narcissism Epidemic*. Her research has been covered in *Time, Newsweek, The New York Times, USA Today*, and the *Washington Post*, and she has been featured on *Today*, NBC *Nightly News, Fox and Friends, Dateline*, and National Public Radio. She received a B.A. and M.A. from the University of Chicago and a Ph.D. from the University of Michigan. She lives in San Diego, California, with her husband and daughters.